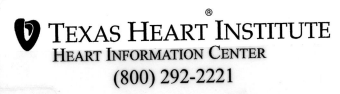

THE MAKING OF THE
PACEMAKER

Celebrating a Lifesaving Invention

Wilson Greatbatch
Inventor of the Pacemaker

Foreword by Seymour Furman, M.D.
Professor of Surgery and Medicine, Albert Einstein College of Medicine

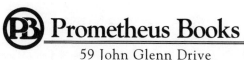 Prometheus Books

59 John Glenn Drive
Amherst, New York 14228-2197

Published 2000 by Prometheus Books

Inquiries should be addressed to
Prometheus Books
59 John Glenn Drive
Amherst, New York 14228-2197
VOICE: 716-691-0133, ext. 207
FAX: 716-564-2711
WWW.PROMETHEUSBOOKS.COM

04 03 02 01 00   5 4 3 2 1

Library of Congress Cataloging-in-Publication Data

Greatbatch, Wilson.
    The making of the pacemaker : celebrating a lifesaving invention / Wilson
Greatbatch.
        p. cm.
    Includes bibliographical references and index.
    ISBN 1-57392-806-2 (cloth : alk. paper)
    1. Cardiac pacemakers—History. I. Title.

RC684.P3 G69 2000
617.4'120645'09—dc21   00-023296
                                                                        CIP

Every attempt has been made to trace accurate ownership of copyrighted material in this book. Errors and omissions will be corrected in subsequent editions,
provided that notification is sent to the publisher.

Printed in the United States of America on acid-free paper

*This book is dedicated to Eleanor,
my loving and long-suffering wife
of fifty-six years,
and to
Warren Dee, John Leslie,
Kenneth Alan, Anne Katherine,
and Peter Neville (1958–1998).*

Contents

Acknowledgments

Of course there would be no book without the past help and compassionate mentoring of Drs. William C. Chardack and Andrew A. Gage.

Also, I must recognize the services of Prometheus Books and my editor, Tara Potzler. Thanks are due to Drs. Bernard Piersma, Steven Calhoun, and Frederick Shannon of the Houghton (New York) College chemistry department where much of the experimental electrode work in chapter 3 was accomplished (in a science building built with pacemaker royalties).

Foreword

by Seymour Furman, M.D.

O n September 10, 1958, the Rockefeller University in New York City sponsored a conference, "Artificial Pacemakers and Artificial Prosthesis," during which many of the major American authorities in cardiac stimulation, cardiac electrophysiology, and the fledgling specialty of medical electronics met to decide on what the future of cardiac pacing might be and the direction it might take. Under the general direction of Vladimir Zworykin of RCA (Radio Corporation of America), an inventor of television, and Carl Berkley, the director of the Division of Medical Electronics of the Rockefeller University, a conference transcript was prepared and finally published in 1993.[1] They were prescient in believing that medical electronics, even as it then existed in a rudimentary form, had a major role to play in medical diagnosis and therapeutics. It had long been known that an electrical stimulus to a muscle would cause a contraction. Some of those present at the conference had demonstrated that when the heart contracted, unlike skeletal muscle (e.g., the muscle of the arms and legs), it seemed to contract in a fashion approximating the normal.

The AV (atrioventricular) conduction system of the heart had been

Seymour Furman, M.D., introduced the technique of transvenous cardiac pacing and demonstrated its long term ability to control heart rate and later the technique of transtelephone monitoring of pacemaker function. He founded and is editor-in-chief of PACE (Pacing and Clinical Electrophysiology), the foremost journal of cardiac pacing and electrical cardiac stimulation. He was a cofounder of NASPE (North American Society of Pacing and Electrophysiology), the premier world organization of this discipline, and his name has been associated with the frontiers of cardiac pacing since its inception in the 1950s. He is Professor of Medicine and Surgery at the Albert Einstein College of Medicine in New York.

discovered and mapped and its function determined during the last years of the nineteenth and the early years of the twentieth centuries[2,3,4]. While much remained to be discovered, and still does, much was known about the cardiac conduction system and the sequence of muscular and chamber contraction. It was known that atrial contraction participated in ventricular filling and that ventricular contraction propelled the blood throughout the body. It had also been observed that the heart stopped beating on occasion and that if it was not promptly restarted, it would then not return to coordinated contraction, and that death resulted.[5] Less clearly, ventricular fibrillation and tachycardia had been recognized,[6] but the comprehension of the extent of their occurrence and the consequent impact on cardiac health awaited the widespread use of Holter monitoring (invented during 1940) in which the patient's electrocardiograph (ECG) is recorded continuously during normal activities over a prolonged period.[7] The recording of the ECG by Waller in 1887[8] and more completely by Einthoven[9] in 1895 had allowed the cardiac electrical activity to be recorded from the body surface. Previously, cardiac activity had been documented by pressure recordings of arterial or venous pulse waves at a peripheral pulse or in the neck at the external jugular vein. It had become progressively more clear that muscular contraction (including cardiac) and electrical activity were closely intertwined.

From 1900 through the 1940s, the new ECG demonstrated the results of the loss of normal cardiac impulse formation or conduction from the atrium to the ventricle via the recently discovered AV conduction system.[10] Resultant periods of asystole (absence of a heart beat) or of a slow (thirty to forty-five beats per minute) and inefficient rate led to heart failure and death. Another possibility was episodic rapid and irregular beating which hardly expelled blood and might cause instantaneous death.[11] Medications, administered intravenously, orally, or sublingually (beneath the tongue, to be absorbed by a moist mucous membrane surface) had been evaluated, and while several had had a modest effect, they were largely without value, especially for long term management.[12] The condition of AV block and asystole with syncope was essentially untreatable. Before the turn of the century the dissociation of atrium from ventricle with associated syncope (loss of consciousness) had been named the Stokes-Adams syndrome after the two Irish physicians who in 1824 and 1854 identified the syndrome of slow heart rates, syncope, and eventual sudden death as all related to cardiac malfunction.[13] (On the European continent the syndrome is referred to as Morgagni-Adams-Stokes after the great Italian physician who described another case, before Stokes or Adams, which he considered epilepsy and not as clearly associated with the heart.[14]) Laboratory electrophysiologists had demonstrated at the beginning of the twentieth century and thereafter that electricity could be used to stimulate the heart.[15] It had not been demonstrated that consistent, reliable, and normally rhythmic contraction, mimicking normal cardiac beating, could result from electrical stimulation.

Several efforts at developing a cardiac stimulator to terminate "cardiac arrest" were made, though "cardiac arrest" was not clearly defined or understood. In 1929 a single, apparently successful effort was made in Australia.[16] In 1930 Albert S. Hyman in New York City had developed a resuscitation device which he named "pacemaker," and he described the attempted resuscitation of several people.[17] His device was independently manufactured and evaluated in Germany and found wanting.[18] Hyman was, however, largely disregarded and did not participate in the Rockefeller University conference. Transvenous catheter atrial pacing in the experimental animal had been achieved by Bigelow and colleagues in Toronto in 1949–50, and a possible attempt at clinical atrial pacing with a catheter for acute onset of complete heart block had been unsuccessful, and the procedure was abandoned.[19] In 1952 Paul Zoll in Boston had invented a transcutaneous pacemaker to be used during emergency asystole. He achieved medical and public recognition and demonstrated the clinical application of pacing in the management of heart block and cardiac arrest.[20] The achievement motivated all of the later developments in cardiac pacing, though Zoll himself hardly moved beyond the transcutaneous approach.

Events were, however, moving so rapidly that some achievements had not yet been published. The Rockefeller University conference provided an incomplete review of the state of knowledge. As can be expected, experts propounded their views of what might be expected of electrical stimulation of the heart, how and where it might be applied therapeutically, and what electrical devices might be useful in its application. Investigators from outside of the United States did not participate so that achievements already in place were not included and accomplishments by those yet without a reputation were also not presented. By the late 1950s the concept of an implantable pacemaker was being seriously considered, though even among the Rockefeller University group the nature of the condition and therefore its proper management was not clearly understood. A major issue was whether continuous or potentially continuous stimulation or episodic stimulation was required. That issue itself was not resolved during the conference.

Aubrey Leatham and Geoffrey Davies in London had already used an external pacemaker with the ability to begin pacing after several seconds without a spontaneous heartbeat and to stop pacing when a spontaneous beat returned.[21] Some presenters at the conference proposed an implantable device for long-term management of Stokes-Adams syndrome. These researchers were opposed to episodic transcutaneous stimulation, as needed, because it was painful and caused skin burns due to the need of 100–150 volts output. It was espoused by Zoll, one of only three with actual clinical experience who attended the conference. In 1957 Earl Bakken, who was at the conference, had invented an external, battery operated pacemaker for use after cardiac surgery.[22] It was never intended for implantation, but rather to stimulate the myocardium via stainless steel wires, and then for a maximum duration of several weeks.

For example, cardiac arrest, during a surgical procedure, was not clearly distinguished from asystole associated with complete heart block and the Stokes-Adams syndrome. Those with clinical experience recognized that stainless steel myocardial suture electrodes used until that time exhibited increasing thresholds, with increased electrical requirements to maintain cardiac response, so that after a period of days or weeks direct myocardial stimulation was unsuccessful. No conceivable implanted pulse generator of that era could cope with the problem. The symposium reviewed the appropriate pacing rate, whether atrial synchrony was desirable for maximum cardiac efficiency, and other issues of cardiac output. Zoll emphasized his external pacing technique, a radio frequency stimulator he was in the process of developing, and the problem of continually rising myocardial stimulation thresholds, with only several weeks of continuous pacing, in a dog. Hellerstein[23] strongly supported atrial synchrony while Zoll, clearly the most prominent pacemaker researcher, believed it to be of little value. While the concept of an implantable pulse generator was discussed and supported by Berkley, Weirich, and Hellerstein, support for a portable, external, transcutaneous stimulator for episodic emergency use was strong. The design of a potential implantable device was stated possibly to be "electrical, mechanical, or chemical."

Looming over the deliberations about an implantable device was the issue of the power source. The Hyman pacemaker of 1930 was powered by manually cranking a magneto (DC generator). Its later manufactured version was powered by primary cells, though the device and its design specifications were lost during the Second World War. The experimental pacemaker built by Hopps for use in Toronto was line powered, as were the Zoll and the Davies and Leatham transcutaneous pacemakers. In 1958 Jorge Reynolds[24] in Bogota, Colombia, designed a pacemaker with a vacuum tube circuit which stimulated the heart with myocardial wires. It was powered by a six-volt lead acid battery. None of these sources allowed the patient significant movement and certainly were inappropriate for implantation.

The problem of how to implant a power source with a practical lifetime persisted. Three possibilities existed. One was the use of an implanted rechargeable (secondary) cell; nickel-cadmium was the only variety available. The second was the use of primary cells, intending that the implanted primary cell-powered pulse generator would have sufficient lifetime to be practical. The mercury-zinc oxide primary cell was invented during the Second World War for military use by Samuel Ruben[25] and was the only possibility for such use. The third was the then recently described transmission of electrical power by radio frequency (RF) or induction so that power would be derived from outside of the body and transmitted to an implanted receiver attached to electrodes.[26] In the event of radio frequency transmission, inexpensive carbon-zinc primary cells could be (and were) used and replaced as frequently as necessary. Radio-frequency transmission of energy to an implanted receiver was a popular means of pacing with at least five systems reaching clinical utilization made by Abrams,[27] Barr,[28] Cammilli,[29] Davies,[30] Glenn,[31] Holswade,[32] Suma and Togawa,[33] and others. Some were used before and others after the advent of the first fully implantable pacemaker.

As the wireless transmission of radio frequency or inductive energy is inefficient, the smallest distance between transmitting coil and receiver was required. Each radio-frequency system suffered from the same difficulties—decoupling of the transmitting coil from the receiving element, wetting and other damage to the external pulse generator, incursion of water into the receiving element, and the need for continual and frequent replacement of batteries. All electrode/leads, including those implanted with the radio frequency receiver, transcutaneous wire, and those attached to an implantable pulse generator, were vulnerable to flexion fracture, corrosion (if not a noble metal, such as platinum), and polarization with rising thresholds. Indeed, rising thresholds were so frequently and consistently observed by early investigators as to be considered a part of myocardial stimulation and a major impediment to long term stimulation.

Events were, however, moving so quickly that most of those present (Zoll and Bakken excepted) had contributed little of permanence to the field. Transvenous pacing, already accomplished in New York (the city of the conference) with demonstrated effectiveness, was not mentioned.[34] Neither William Glenn of New Haven nor William Chardack and Wilson Greatbatch of Buffalo, New York (all geographically proximate), or other overseas workers such as Cammilli or Leatham and Davies, attended. Bakken and his fledgling company Medtronic had, in 1957, invented a functional external battery-operated pacemaker at the request of C. Walton Lillehei, one of the founders of open heart surgery.[35] He had found that repair of some congenital cardiac lesions caused heart block and that safe management required a pacemaker with a power source independent of the fallible general municipal electrical grid.

Eventually three teams were in the process of developing a wholly implantable device which each designed to be powered by mercury-zinc cells. The earliest group was headed by Chardack, Gage, and Greatbatch of Buffalo, New York,[36] and later Zoll of Boston[37] and Kantrowitz of Brooklyn.[38] Wilson Greatbatch, an electrical engineer, had worked in the research laboratory at Cornell University in Ithaca, New York, where he had participated in projects involving mammalian neurologic and muscular stimulation. He had begun to conceive of the possibility of a primary cell powered implantable device for long-term stimulation. A major and most important decision was that the pulse generator and the power source would be wholly implanted to avoid the difficulties of radio-frequency power transmission. Rechargeability was also rejected. This change in direction from what had gone before was critical to the eventual success of his design.

The decision that the pulse generator would be wholly implantable, requiring no additional management and the erroneous calculation that a mercury-zinc powered pulse generator would have a duration of some five years before exhaustion, were central to the success of the design. As in so many other instances, one can only wonder how the effort would have progressed if all of the eventually manifest technical difficulties had been considered as the pacemaker was being developed. He and Drs. William Chardack and Andrew Gage eventually began a project for the development of an implantable pacemaker with Greatbatch working in a shed on his property.

The first forty-five patients had pulse generators powered by ten mercury-zinc cells (13.5 volts) and a simple two-transistor circuit.[39] The group accomplished the first clinically successful complete implant of leads and pulse generator, as the second stage of a two-stage procedure, on June 6, 1960. The Zoll group completed their first implant on November 7, 1960, and the Kantrowitz group May 5, 1961. With the Chardack-Greatbatch implant, and their subsequent agreement with Medtronic for manufacture, the era of implantable cardiac pacing began.

The pulse generator design was based on the availability of the newly introduced transistor and the epoxy resin in which the circuit could be encased. It was also known that electrical stimuli could cause the ventricles to contract and that a cardiac contraction would closely mimic a normal heart beat and expel blood effectively. Construction of the pacemaker was also based on what was not known. It was not known that the calculation of the power contained in the cell selected to power the pulse generator was substantially incorrect, and it was also not known that though incorrect, the pulse generator would have sufficient durability to function long enough to demonstrate the feasibility of the approach. It was already known that the Hunter-Roth electrode, introduced for direct myocardial stimulation with an external pulse generator, would function for a prolonged period necessary to demonstrate the viability of the technique. What was not clear was that bare stainless steel wire electrodes would almost certainly not function long and that flat surface electrodes might function for the long term.

Available information in the medical literature, which did not seem to influence the design, was the possibility of creating a pulse generator which would respond to a spontaneous heart beat by withholding a pacemaker stimulus, a design which had already been described by Davies. Successful long term cardiac stimulation by an endocardial electrode[40] was disregarded in pursuing a more traditional approach to placement of the myocardial electrodes by thoracotomy. Still, it was known that stimulation threshold tended to rise and that sufficient rise would cause cessation of pacing. A generous output of 13.5 volts was selected, well above the minimum needed to stimulate the heart, and soon after the first pulse generator, a mechanism (the pig tail), was added to allow intervention and increase pulse generator output if necessary.

As with every introduction of a new concept, the implantable pacemaker was a combination of brilliant analysis and foresight and possibly a degree of fortuitous selection. Technology and techniques selected and others disregarded which might have changed implementation and rejection of real or imagined problems might have stalled the effort or changed its direction. Other previously implemented approaches to implantation, with the rechargeable cell or radio-frequency transmission, had employed bare wire electrodes buried in the myocardium. These were characterized by rapid increase in stimulation threshold and early inability of the system to continue effectively stimulating the heart. The effect on the success of these systems of inadequate electrodes has not been fully considered. At the time of implantation of the Chardack-Greatbatch pacemaker, experience with the Bakken external pacemaker and the Hunter-Roth bipolar platform electrode suggested that long term stable pacing could be anticipated. That electrode availability was fortuitous. Its use with the new pulse generator immediately provided the ability for relatively long term stable pacing. Other electrode options were disregarded such as transvenous pacing, which by mid–1960 had a successful published experience. Had such an approach been selected in 1960 rather than five years later, modern cardiac pacing, an implanted pulse generator, and a transvenous right ventricular lead would have been in place in 1960. That combination went to Hans Lagergren in Stockholm in 1963.[41] Had the possibility of return of conduction or the need to manage spontaneous ventricular ectopy been recognized, a pulse generator which stimulated in the absence of spontaneous beating and ceased while spontaneous beating occurred, the demand or VVI approach could have been developed. Such capability had been described by Davies and Leatham in 1956 and was incorporated into an external stimulator, manufactured by Firth-Cleveland in Wales, United Kingdom.

Still, none of these approaches, which can always be anticipated in any truly original and groundbreaking innovation, should detract from the great accomplishment. Unlike those who did not fully recognize their accomplishments or did not recognize that research and development are different from device manufacture, Greatbatch, Chardack, and Gage patented their device and undertook an agreement for manufacture with the then ten-year-old firm Medtronic, Inc. of Minneapolis. That agreement effectively began the modern medical device industry.

Twelve years later Greatbatch made his second great contribution to implantable devices. In 1958–1960 he selected the most suitable power source available, the mercury-zinc cell, to power the device. Time and use soon demonstrated the inadequacy of that power source to provide long term pacing consistent with patient needs. It soon became evident that despite a design estimate of five years function, the Ruben mercury-zinc cell battery, in a pacemaker pulse generator, never exceeded an average of eighteen to twenty-four months. These nonhermetically sealed cells leaked potassium hydroxide and destroyed the pulse generator circuit while the cell's evolution of hydrogen during electricity production precluded hermetic sealing. The cell's continued function depended on the body's ability to absorb those small and harmless amounts of hydrogen. The circuit soon swam in a pool of 100 percent humidity.[42] Last, but certainly not least, the cell had a rapid internal discharge (shelf-life) compared to implant needs. About 10 percent of the capacity of a Ruben mercury-zinc cell was lost annually, at body temperature, even if not evolving electricity. Those problems never did allow the successful long term use of Ruben mercury-zinc cells for implantable devices.

While pulse generator shortcomings were apparent to both physicians and industry, the changes made were in reducing pulse generator output and circuit efficiency, anticipating that lower output would result in longer duration. That approach was minimally successful. Greatbatch demonstrated that despite changes in circuit design and increase in efficiency, all of the competing pulse generator designs had essentially the same longevity so that that approach was largely fruitless. When a new cell was invented in 1968 and held out the possibility of low level prolonged service life, he evaluated it as a possibility.[43] The lithium iodine cell had double the output voltage of the mercury cell (2.8 volts versus 1.35 volts), a large capacity, i.e., 3 ampere-hours versus 1 ampere hour, did not evolve gas during electricity production, and had low internal discharge. It could be hermetically sealed and incorporated in a pulse generator which could itself be hermetically sealed. Greatbatch was a proponent of the lithium iodine battery and with that the modern, long duration, hermetically sealed pulse generator. In the process a new pacemaker manufacturer was founded, Cardiac Pacemakers Inc. (CPI), to manufacture pulse generators powered by the lithium iodine cell.

When association with physicians was necessary to break truly new ground and invent and then implant a pulse generator, Greatbatch did that. Later when what was needed was the introduction of an entirely new means of making an implantable pulse generator, he was dealing with an industry he had helped create and that was to varying degrees receptive to the new power source. The older manufacturers were, as a group, cautious about adopting the new power source, possibly because of a need to be certain of its effectiveness and safety, possibly because an investment in mercury-zinc, and possibly because of short-sightedness. But the entrepreneurial groups leaped onto the new power source, designed pulse generators, and made them work. One such manufacturer was LEM in Italy, and the second, the newly formed CPI. In the process Greatbatch eventually destroyed each of the other competing power sources: mercury-zinc, nickel-cadmium, and nuclear in the form of plutonium or promethium isotopes. Following the introduction of the lithium-iodine cell, four competitive lithium anode cells were introduced: lithium-lead, lithium silver chromate, lithium thionyl chloride, and lithium cupric sulfide. Only the last has proved to be durable, with some pulse generators functioning ten to twelve years after being placed into service. Nevertheless, all four are no longer used to power implantable pulse generators. Only the lithium iodine cell, introduced by Greatbatch, survived.

That's quite a record of accomplishment.

NOTES

1. K. Jeffrey, Conference on Artificial Pacemakers and Cardiac Prosthesis, Sponsored by The Medical Electronics Center of the Rockefeller Institute, 1958. *PACE* 16 (1993): 1445-82.

2. W. His Jr., "Die Thetigkeit des embryonalen Herzens und deren Bedeutung fur die Lehre von der Herzbewegung beim Erwacsenen." *Arch Med Klin Leipzig* 14 (1893): 14-49.

3. S. Tawara, *Das Reizleitungssystem des Saugetierherens*. Gustav Fischer Jena, 1906.

4. T. Lewis, B. S. Oppenheimer, and A. Oppenheimer, "The Site of Origin of the Mammalian Heart Beat; The Pacemaker in the Dog." *Heart* 2 (1910-1911): 147-69.

5. J. Erlanger, "On the Physiology of Heart-block in Mammals, with Especial Reference to Causation of Stokes-Adams Disease. Part I. Observations On an Instance of Heart Block in Man." *J Exp Med* 7 (1905): 676-724.

6. L. Gallavardin and A. Berard, "Un cas de fibrillation ventricularire au cours des accidents syncopaux du Stokes-Adams." *Arch Mal Coeur* 17 (1924): 18–20.

7. N. Holter, "A New Method for Heart Studies: Continuous Electrocardiography of Active Subjects Over Long Periods is Now Practical." *Science* 134 (1961): 1214–20.

8. A. D. Waller, "A Demonstration on Man of Electromotive Changes Accompanying the Heart's Beat." *J Physiol* 8 (1887): 229.

9. W. Einthoven, "Ueber die Form des menschlichen Electrocardiogramms." *Pfluger's Arch* 60 (1895): 101–23.

10. J. Parkinson, C. Papp, and W. Evans, "The Electrocardiogram of the Stokes-Adams Attack." *Brit Heart J* 3 (1941): 171–99.

11. S. P. Schwartz and A. Jezer, "Action of Quinine and Quinidine Sulphate on Patients with Transient Ventricular Fibrillation." *Amer Heart J* 9 (1934): 792.

12. A. E. Cohn and S. A. Levine, "The Beneficial Effects of Barium Chloride on Adams-Stokes Disease." *Arch Intern Med*, Chicago 36 (1925): 1–12.

13. H. Huchard, "Le maladie de Stokes-Adams." *Bull Med*, Paris 4 (1890): 937–40.

14. G. Morgagni, "Letter the Ninth, Which Treats Epilepsy." In *De Sedibus et Causis Morborium*, 1761. (*The Seats and Causes of Diseases*, trans. by Benjamin Alexander, London: Millar & Cadell, 1762, p. 92.)

15. J. A. MacWilliam, "Electrical Stimulation of the Heart in Man." *Brit M J* 1 (1889): 348–50.

16. H. G. Mond, J. G. Sloman, and R. H. Edwards, "The First Pacemaker." *PACE* 5 (1982): 278–82.

17. A. S. Hyman, "Resuscitation of the Stopped Heart By Intracardiac Therapy." *Arch Intern Med* 46 (1930): 553–68.

18. S. Koeppen, "Untersuchungen über die Wirksamkeit von Wiederbelebungsmassnahmen bei Experimenteller Erstickung." *Klin Wochen* 14 (1935): 1131–33.

19. W. G. Bigelow, "The Pacemaker Story: A Cold Heart Spinoff." *PACE* 10 (1987): 142–50.

20. P. M. Zoll, "Resuscitation of the Heart in Ventricular Standstill By External Electric Stimulation." *N Eng J Med* 247 (1952): 768–71.

21. A. Leatham, P. Cook, and J. G. Davies, "External Electric Stimulator for Treatment of Ventricular Standstill." *Lancet* 2 (1956): 1185–89.

22. W. L. Weirich, M. Paneth, V. L. Gott, and C. W. Lillehei, "Control of Complete Heart Block By Use of an Artificial Pacemaker and a Myocardial Electrode." *Circ Res* 6 (1958): 410–15.

23. H. K. Hellerstein, D. Shaw, and I. M. Liebow, "An Extracorporeal Electronics Bypass of the A-V Node." *J Lab & Clin Med* 36 (1950): 833.

24. J. Reynolds, "The Early History of Cardiac Pacing in Colombia." *PACE* 11 (1988): 355–61.

25. S. Ruben, "Sealed Zinc-Mercuric Oxide Cells for Implantable Cardiac Pacemakers." In *Advances in Cardiac Pacemakers*, ed. S. Furman. *Ann NY Acad Sci.* 167 (1969): 627–34.

26. M. Verzeano, R. G. Webb Jr., and M. Kelly, "Radio Control of Ventricular Contraction in Experimental Heart Block." *Science* 128 (1958): 1003.

27. L. D. Abrams, W. A. Hudson, and R. Lightwood, "A Surgical Approach to the Management of Heart-block Using an Inductive Coupled Artificial Cardiac Pacemaker." *Lancet* 1 (1960): 1372–74.

28. I. M. Barr, S. Yerushalmi, L. Blieden, and H. N. Neufeld, "Endocardial Radio-frequency Pacemaking." *Israel J Med Sci* 1 (1965): 1018–21.

29. L. Cammilli, R. Pozzi, G. Drago, G. Pizzichi, and G. De Saint-Pierre, "Remote Heart Stimulation By Radio-frequency for Permanent Rhythm Control in the Morgagni-Adams-Stokes Syndrome." *Surgery* 52 (1962): 765–76.

30. J. G. Davies, "Artificial Cardiac Pacemakers for the Long-term Treatment of Heart Block." *J Brit Inst Radio Engr* 24 (1962): 453.

31. W. W. L. Glenn, A. Mauro, E. Longo, P. H. Lavietes, and F. J. MacKay, "Remote Stimulation of the Heart by Radio-frequency Transmission." *N Eng J Med* 261 (1959): 948–51.

32. G. R. Holswade and C. Linardos, "Induction Pacemaker for Control of Complete Heart Block." *J Thorac Cardiovasc Surg* 44 (1962): 246–52.

33. M. Suma, Y. Fujimori, T. Mitsui, M. Hori, K. Asano, S. Kimoto, T. Togawa, and J. Nagumo, "Direct Induction Pacemaker." *Digest of the 6th International Conference on Medical Electronic and Biological Engineering*, Tokyo, 1965: 96.

34. S. Furman and J. B. Schwedel, "An Intracardiac Pacemaker for Stokes-Adams Seizures." *N Eng J Med* 261 (1959): 943–48.

35. C. W. Lillehei, V. L. Gott, P. C. Hodges, D. M. Long, and E. E. Bakken, "Transistor Pacemaker for Treatment of Complete Atrioventricular Dissociation." *JAMA* 172 (1960): 2006–10.

36. W. Chardack, A. A. Gage, and W. Greatbatch, "A Transistorized, Self-contained Implantable Pacemaker for the Long-term Correction of Complete Heart Block." *Surgery* 48 (1960): 643–54.

37. P. M. Zoll, H. A. Frank, L. R. Zarsky, A. J. Linenthal, and A. H. Belgard, "Long-term Electrical Stimulation of the Heart for Stokes-Adams Disease." *Ann Surg* 154 (1961): 330–46.

38. A. Kantrowitz, R. Cohen, H. Raillard, J. Schmidt, and D. S. Feldman, "The Treatment of Complete Heart Block with an Implanted Controllable Pacemaker." *Surg Gynec Obstet* 115 (1962): 415–20.

39. W. M. Chardack, A. A. Gage, A. J. Federico, G. Schimert, and W. Greatbatch, "Clinical Experience with an Implantable Pacemaker." *Ann NY Acad Sci* 111 (1964): 1075–92.

40. H. Siddons and J. G. Davies, "A New Technique for Internal Cardiac Pacing." *Lancet* 2 (1963): 1204–1205.

41. H. Lagergren, L. Johansson, J. Landegren, and O. Edhag, "One Hundred Cases of Treatment for Adams-Stokes Syndrome with Permanent Intravenous Pacemaker." *J Thorac and Cardiovasc Surg* 50 (1965): 710–14.

42. G. F. O. Tyers and R. R. Brownlee, "The Non-hermetically Sealed Pacemaker Myth, or Navy-Ribicoff 22,000—FDA-Weinberger 0." *J Thorac Cardiovasc Surg* 1976; 71:253–54.

43. A. Schneider, J. Moser, T. H. E. Webb, and J. E. Desmond, "A New High Energy Density Cell with a Lithium Anode." *Proc US Army Signal Corps Power Sources Conf*, Atlantic City, N.J., 1970.

Introduction

This book documents the development and critical follow-up years of the implantable cardiac pacemaker (U.S. Patent 3,057,356). Use in an experimental animal took place in May, 1958, and its successful use in a patient occurred on April 7, 1960 ("successful" defined here as demonstration of over a year's continual use). The implantable cardiac pacemaker was the first self-powered prosthetic device ever to be totally implanted in the human body to permanently replace a lost physiological function. It has been suggested that the invention and successful use of this device launched the implantable medical device industry.

Pacemaker technology has since undergone great advances. However, lithium battery chemistry and the electrochemical polarization of physiological electrodes described here remain state-of-the art technologies.

The twenty-fifth anniversary of our first pacemaker implantation in an experimental animal was in 1983. At that time I wrote a book on our years of work. It was privately published, and 1,500 copies were distributed to friends and colleagues.

Now, at the beginning of a new millennium, it seems appropriate to professionally reproduce this book in hard cover to serve as a historical document for those who shared in pacemaker development as well as for those dedicated to improving future health care worldwide.

Some updating has been done, but most of it has been left in its original form as a historical record. (An obvious exception is chapter 11 on nuclear fusion.) Thus the reader should go to other more modern sources for such things as multichamber pacing and electrophysiology. The book is divided into twelve chapters. The first chapter is largely history and nostalgia. Occasional regressions into "The Way It Was" describe interesting events or interesting people with whom the author came into contact. The last chapter is essentially a sermon to young engineers as to how to get yourself accepted into full collaboration with the medical profession.

The intervening chapters are largely technical treatises on electrodes, power sources, and infection control. A lengthy chapter is devoted to the electrochemical mechanism of cardiac electrodes on the heart (electrochemical polarization of physiological electrodes). Electricity flows through wires by means of electron flow, but through fluids and tissue by ion flow. To get an ion from an electron requires a chemical reaction, with a different reaction at the positive electrode than at the negative electrode. The reaction takes place within a millionth of an inch of the surface of the metal, and the coupling reaction which takes place depends entirely on the electrode metal used. Thus, the same pacemaker driving the same heart may go through four different books on electrochemistry, depending on the electrode metal used. One reaction, that of a small-area stainless steel positive electrode, is a corrosion reaction. Hardly desirable in a cardiac electrode!

I hope you enjoy reading my book as much as I have in writing it, and in reliving those exciting years.

Wilson Greatbatch, FACC, FIEEE, P.E.

1

EARLY PEOPLE
AND EARLY SYSTEMS

INTRODUCTION

May 7, 2000, marked the forty-second anniversary of the first implantable cardiac pacemaker. On that day, Dr. William C. Chardack, Dr. Andrew Gage, and I implanted the first self-powered implantable cardiac pacemaker in an experimental animal.[1]

In October, later the same year, Dr. Ake Senning and chemical engineer Rune Elmqvist in Stockholm attempted the first human clinical implant. It worked for three hours. A replacement worked eight days, after which the patient went unstimulated for some three years.[2] The patient, Mr. Larson, was still alive in 2000. Senning and Elmqvist deserve much credit for this early attempt at a human implant, which was accomplished under very adverse circumstances. At a luncheon in Stockholm, Dr. Elmqvist told me that he built these first two prototypes in the cellar of his apartment. I am impressed by how much of the early pacemaker history emerged from garages, barns, and cellars. In 1960, our group accomplished the first clinically successful implant.[3,4]

In 1958, we foresaw an optimistic annual usage of about 10,000 pacemakers per year. In a remarkably short time, the implantable pacemaker became the treatment of choice for complete heart block with Stokes-Adam syndrome. Today, more than forty years later, pacemakers have assumed forms and functions that we never dreamed of, and the world pacemaker market is well over 600,000 units per year.

It seems fitting therefore to sit down and document everything that I can remember about the people and events, about the components and designs, and about all that happened to us in those forty-two years. It is a very personal record, subject to personal bias, largely written in the first person. I have also chosen to inject flashbacks or side trips of "how it was." These may well be out of place, but this is my book and I'm going to do it my way. I know I have missed dozens of friends who had a part in our work, and I have undoubtedly short-changed the work of others in these four decades. For this, my apologies. I can only hope that what I have put down will be entertaining to some, nostalgic for others, and perhaps somewhere, someone might be saved from making a mistake that we already made and wrote about. If an expert is one who has made most of the mistakes, we probably qualify. The wise man is the one who doesn't make them twice. We've missed here, too, occasionally.

It's been a fantastic forty-two years. My heartfelt thanks go to all those who were a part of it. Few engineers are given the chance to change history. The Good Lord has presented us with this opportunity no less than three times. The invention of the implantable cardiac pacemaker is described in chapter 1. The introduction of the clinically implantable lithium battery is in chapter 4, and our participation in helium-3 nuclear fusion energy can be found in chapter 11.

I hope you enjoy my book.

EARLY PEOPLE AND EARLY SYSTEMS

Autobiographical Notes 1930–1950

I have five children. My four sons are all mechanically inclined. They handle metal well, and three of them work beautifully with wood. None of them has the slightest interest in electronics. I have always wondered why. Electricity and electronics have always fascinated me. I think it was the mystery of it. Something was happening that you couldn't see, or feel, or hear. You needed a meter or an oscilloscope or at least a neon bulb to detect it, and then you had to interpret what the reading meant. I know I was thoroughly hooked early in my teens when I built my first two-tube short-wave receiver and listened to London, England, on a coil I had wound myself. I think I was sixteen when I passed the test for my radio amateur's license (W8QBD). I was also very active in Boy Scouts and joined the Sea Scout Radio Division which had a station (W8QBU) at the Buffalo (New York) Sea Scout Base at the foot of Porter Avenue, next to the New York State Naval Militia in Buffalo. During the 1937 New England hurricane our station received a Red Cross citation for handling emergency traffic. We were quite proud.

THE WAY IT WAS

I spent many weekends at the Sea Scout Base sailing, rowing, or talking over the transmitter to other "hams." One evening I put the rig on the air and was amazed to hear some stations on the East coast trying to get emergency messages out. The 1937 hurricane that devastated New England had hit the coast. I started taking the traffic and passing it westward to other ham stations in Ontario or Ohio. Several of the other operators in our club heard me on the air and came down to help. We kept our station on the air for twenty-six hours, passing messages back and forth. We were cited by the Red Cross for this work.

*   *   *

As Sea Scouts, we used to row a one-ton, five-oared whaleboat several miles out to Waverly Shoals in Lake Erie. The boat was designed for rescues at sea in the heaviest weather and was steered by an oar rather than by a rudder, which would have hung out of the water most of the time in a heavy sea. It was horribly hard work but we loved it. One Sunday in Santiago (Cuba) harbor, our division of four destroyers held a one-mile whaleboat race, a navy tradition. Our ship entered our Sea Scout crew and we won the race. The prize was a carton of cigarettes for each man in the crew, but none of us smoked!

Our club had social activities as well, and a group of the girls that we went with formed an informal auxiliary. They made curtains for our radio shack (ugh!). They called their "sorority" MAD, which stood for "Men Are Dogs." Most of the guys finally married most of the girls, as I did, too, eventually.

In 1939–1940 some of us joined the naval reserve unit next door. The fact that we had an amateur radio license qualified us for a non-commissioned officer's rating. We took part in naval radio drills and went to sea two weeks each summer. In 1939 we sailed out of New York on a heavy cruiser (the *U.S.S. Vincennes*, later sunk in WW II) and had a chance to see the World's Fair there that year. In 1940 we sailed to Guantanamo and Santiago in Cuba on a four-stack destroyer.

By 1940 the international situation was deteriorating and our naval reserve unit was called up for one year's active duty, but I got out five years later. One by one, our club radio operators went into service, but other new members came up to take their place. By the end of the war, our club had put more than fifty radio operators into military service. Three men later became professors of electrical engineering and about two dozen went into careers as radio technicians, some in government service with the Federal Aviation Administration (FAA), some into police radio, and others into private industry. Those were quite some accomplishments for a group of Boy Scouts. Sometimes I think we handled our teenagers better in those days.

My own navy time consisted of repairing electronic equipment on a destroyer tender (the *U.S.S. Melville*), "pounding brass" as a navy radio operator on merchant ships in convoy to Iceland, teaching in a navy radar school at Ward Island, Corpus Christi, Texas, and finally flying in combat as a rear gunner off an aircraft carrier (the *U.S.S. Monterey**) in dive bombers and torpedo bombers. Ours was a small nine-plane squadron, but we used twenty-seven airplanes in six months of combat. A third of our crew was killed.

With WW II over in 1945, I returned to Buffalo with my new bride, worked a year as an installer-repairman with the New York Telephone Company, and then decided to register in the School of Electrical Engineering at Cornell University in Ithaca, New York.

THE WAY IT WAS

They wouldn't admit me at Cornell. There was room in the school, but no housing for nonresident students. So I went out to Danby, six miles south of Ithaca, and bought a farm. Then I came back and presented myself as a "resident student." I got in.

Cornell was wonderful! After all that time in the dive-bombers, it was such a joy to wander around the campus, to go to class and to learn something, to be a part of the great tradition of all that had gone before. I was so grateful. I have repeatedly and vainly tried to imbue my children with the kind of appreciation that I had, just for the opportunity to sit, and hear, and learn. I don't think I ever got this across to them. Maybe you have to come straight down two miles with the "ack-ack" of gunfire bursting all around you to appreciate the change.

Cornell has always stressed breadth of background. Thus we got enough math to qualify us as high school math teachers, and more physics and chemistry than most other schools ever provide. I still remember and use some of the lectures we heard on patent law and on being an expert witness. My work since then has been mostly outside of my specific training as an electronic circuit designer. The breadth of

---

*Former President Ford was our deck officer.

background Cornell gave me has enabled me to branch out when necessary into nuclear physics, electrochemical polarization of physiological
electrodes, battery chemistry, the physics of welding, and the countless
other things I have had to do in the past decades to keep our corporate
heads above water.

My first contact with medical electronics came during my under-
graduate days at Cornell. I was a "GI Bill" student, my only honor being
that I had more children than anyone else in the class (three at the
time). To feed my family, I had to double my GI bill income. During one
period I ran the university AM/FM transmitter (WHCU) on weekends.
At other times I worked as an electronics technician, building IF amplifiers for what was later to become the Arecibo radio telescope in Puerto
Rico. One day in an adjacent lab I saw a graduate student, Frank Noble
(later to become head of an electronics laboratory at the National Institutes of Health), measuring the blood pressure in a rat by measuring the
change in tail size as a pulse of blood traversed it. His electronic plethys-
mograph was part of the instrumentation at the Psychology Department's Animal Behavior Farm at Varna, New York, near Ithaca, under
Dr. Urner Liddel. Noble was responsible for checking about one hundred
sheep and goats for heart rate and blood pressure. Dr. Liddel's experiments dealt with conditioned reflex under neurosis. I became intensely
interested, and when Noble left to go with NIH, I inherited his job.

This exposure to Pavlovian psychology was to prove most useful
when we were called on five years later to provide the physiological
telemetry for the space monkeys Sam and Miss Sam launched from
Wallops Island in Virginia by the United States Air Force in their early
space probes.

THE WAY IT WAS

Brown Billy was an old retired goat who loved to eat cigarettes. He had
a venerable history in Pavlovian conditioned reflex, which consisted of
standing in a stall and lifting his right leg when a bell rang, but ignoring
a buzzer signal. Reason: If he ignored a bell signal, he got a mild electrical shock in the rump. One hot summer day, when the pasture was dry,
we electric-fenced a new hayfield and turned the goats into it. Billy had
never seen an electric fence before. He grazed over towards it and finally
got bit by it. He jumped straight up in the air, came down about twenty
feet away, turned, ruefully looked at the fence, and then dutifully raised
his right rear leg.

During the summer of 1951, a pair of New England brain surgeons spent their summer sabbatical at the farm doing experimental brain surgery on the hypothalamus of goats. They were investigating the influence of the hypothalamus on behavior. The surgeons carried their lunches in brown bags, as did I, and noontimes we would sit on the grass in the bright Ithaca sun and talk shop. I learned much practical physiology from them. At times the subject of heart block came up. When they described it, I knew I could fix it, but not with the vacuum tubes and storage batteries we had then.

EARLY HISTORY 1950–1956

I went into aerospace work at Cornell Aeronautical Laboratory (CAL) in Buffalo, keeping all of my previous experiences in my mind and not knowing that Paul Zoll was building his first historic external pacemakers in Boston at that time.

In 1953 we saw our first transistors at CAL. I built some amplifiers with them. In 1956, the first really commercial silicon transistors became available (at $90 each), and I began using them. At the time I was an assistant professor at the University of Buffalo School of Electrical Engineering, but was spending some time with Dr. Simon Rodbard and Dr. Robert Cohn at the Chronic Disease Research Institute on Main Street in Buffalo. Rodbard was interested in fast heart sounds which we recorded off an oscilloscope with a movie camera. I wanted a 1Khz marker oscillator and built one out of a single transistor and a UTC DOT-1 transformer.

THE WAY IT WAS

My marker oscillator used a 10K basebias resistor. I reached into my resistor box for one but misread the colors and got a brown-black-green (one megohm) instead of a brown-black-orange. The circuit started to "squeg" with a 1.8 ms pulse, followed by a one second quiescent interval. During the interval, the transistor was cut off and drew practically no current. I stared at the thing in disbelief and then realized that this was exactly what was needed to drive a heart. I built a few more. For the next five years, most of the world's pacemakers used a blocking oscillator with a UTC DOT-1 transformer, just because I grabbed the wrong resistor.

Neither Cohn nor Rodbard were much interested in pacemakers although both were cardiologists; nor was Dr. Dave Green, a cardiologist at Buffalo General Hospital, another member of our early Professional Group in Medical Electronics (PGME), so I kept looking.

I found little enthusiasm locally in 1958 for an implantable pacemaker. Each medical group I approached said, "Fine idea, but most of these patients die in a year or so. Why don't you work on my project?" Then one day in the spring of 1958, I visited Dr. William Chardack, chief of surgery at the Veterans Administration Hospital in Buffalo.

THE WAY IT WAS

In Buffalo we had the first local chapter in the world of the Institute of Radio Engineers, Professional Group in Medical Electronics (the IRE/ PGME, now the Biomedical Engineering Society of the Institute of Electrical and Electronic Engineers [IEEE]). Every month twenty-five to seventy-five doctors and engineers met for a technical program. We strove to attract equal numbers of doctors and engineers. We had a standing offer to send an engineering team to assist any doctor who had an instrumentation problem. I went with one team to visit Dr. Chardack on a problem dealing with a blood oximeter. Imagine my surprise to find that his assistant was my old high school classmate, Dr. Andrew Gage. We couldn't help Dr. Chardack much with his oximeter problem, but when I broached my pacemaker idea to him, he walked up and down the lab a couple of times, looked at me strangely, and said, "If you can do that, you can save ten thousand lives a year." Three weeks later we had our first model implanted in a dog.

ANIMAL EXPERIMENTATION, 1958

Our experimental work was done on dogs that had been put into complete heart block by occluding the AV (atrioventricular) bundle with a tied suture, as taught by Dr. Starzl. We had no heart-lung machine. The operating team stood poised like runners waiting for the starting gun. Upon a "go" signal, the team occluded the large vessels, opened the heart, occluded the AV bundle with the tied suture, closed the heart, and released the artery, all in about ninety seconds!

We were pretty naive about early pacemaker designs. We thought that wrapping the module in electric tape would seal it. We soon found that any void would fill with fluid and we began to cast our electronics into a solid epoxy block (3M Scotchcast V). Within a year we had worked our survival time up from four hours to four months, and felt ready to start looking for a suitable clinical patient.

The time needed to build the units began taking more of my time than my job would allow. My employer at the time, Ralph Taber of Taber Instrument Corp. in North Tonawanda, New York, was unwilling to jeopardize his million-dollar company on a liability like the pacemaker, especially after Lloyd's of London turned him down on liability insurance. I then made the decision to work full time on the pacemaker and on some astronaut instrumentation that we were building for the early animal space shots.

THE WAY IT WAS

I had $2,000 in cash and enough set aside to feed my family for two years. I put it to the Lord in prayer and felt led to quit all my jobs and devote my time to the pacemaker. I gave the family money to my wife. I then took the $2,000 and went up into my wood-heated barn workshop. In two years I built fifty pacemakers, forty of which went into animals and ten into patients. We had no grant funding and asked for none. The program was successful. We got fifty pacemakers for $2,000. Today, you can't buy one for that.

FIRST CLINICAL USE

During 1960 I handmade dozens of pacemakers, some of which were successfully implanted in ten patients by Dr. Chardack and his associates. Most of the patients were older people in their sixties, seventies, and eighties, typical of the usual heart-block patient. Two, however, were children, and one was a young man who worked in a local rubber factory until he collapsed on the job. His prognosis was grim. After receiving a pacemaker he retrained as a hairdresser, worked full time, and joined a bowling team. He was still alive and well in 1990. It is given to very few engineers to say to a patient, "Pick up thy bed and walk." It is given to us and we appreciate it.

Another patient I remember well was an older woman, also in complete block with Stokes-Adam syndrome. When my local engineering society named me "Engineer of the Year," she came to my award dinner. The news media called her the "Pacemaker Queen." She died in her eighties, after being paced for more than twenty years.

I think one of my first and most gratifying realizations of what a pacemaker could do was in observing the reactions of older people to their grandchildren. When in block, these older people generally didn't have enough blood supply to their brain and couldn't respond quickly to the bantering of the kids. The kids would say, "Well, Grandpa's dottery," and go off about their play. With a pacemaker, Grandpa could snap back at the kids and be in the mainstream again. I think this, more than anything else, changed his life. Now that I am (six times) a grandfather myself, I fully realize the impact of what I saw.

Electrodes were a major problem from the beginning. We first used simple myocardial wires but found long-term thresholds to be unstable. We tried stranded wire, solid wire, silver wire, stainless steel, and orthodontic gold and platinum and its alloys. Our first clinical success was achieved with Medtronic's Hunter-Roth electrode. This electrode had two stainless steel pins perpendicularly supported in a silicone rubber base plate. They eventually failed because of corrosion on the small area anode pin and its lead. By that time Dr. Chardack had developed a myocardial electrode based on a platinum-iridium spring coil. This matured into the Medtronic Model 5814 myocardial electrode which was widely used for many years.

All these designs were myocardial electrodes that required a thoracotomy (an open-chest procedure). The surgical insult plus the general anesthesia resulted in a 10 percent early mortality in these older, at-risk patients. In the meantime, Dr. Seymour Furman at Montefiori Hospital in New York had developed a transvenous approach using an endocardial catheter (inside the heart) for temporary pacing.[5] Chardack combined this approach with a spring coil lead resulting in a permanent endocardial catheter electrode which eventually became the Medtronic 5816/5818 series. A temporary stiff stylet was threaded down the spring coil to control it during insertion.

In Sweden, Dr. Ake Senning, Dr. Hans Lagergren, and the Karolinska Institute group developed a flaccid catheter which utilized a temporary stiff tube around the catheter, rather than a wire through the center, to assist in catheter orientation during insertion. These became very popular in Europe but saw little use in America. One exception was during the extended visit of Prof. C. Crafoord from Karolinska to Dr. Murray Anderson's laboratory at Meyer Memorial Hospital in Buffalo. Unfortunately, we had no contact with their group, which was probably a lost opportunity for some meaningful interaction.

EARLY MEDTRONIC YEARS 1960–1963

We had been aware of Medtronic's work in external, wearable pacemakers, both through Dr. Norman Roth and James Anderson of Medtronic, and through Dr. Chardack's friendship with Dr. C. Walton Lillehei of the University of Minnesota Hospital in Minneapolis. We had learned of silicone rubber and medical adhesive through Norman Roth and, in fact, the first electrodes we used clinically were the Hunter-Roth electrodes, designed by Roth and Dr. Sam Hunter of Minneapolis, and built by Medtronic. At that time, Medtronic was still a very small company located in a garage in Minneapolis. Earl Bakken, the president, was an electrical engineer whose fiancee, Connie, was a medical technician for Dr. Lillehei. While waiting for Connie, Bakken would wander around the lab and occasionally talk shop with Dr. Lillehei.

Dr. Lillehei at that time was doing some of the first open-heart surgery on children. He occasionally ran into cases of complete heart block in children, and Dr. W. Weirich began leaving electrode wires temporarily in place after surgery. After a near catastrophe during which a power failure incapacitated the line-operated stimulators, Bakken decided he could build a wearable, battery-operated stimulator to drive the electrodes. Soon Medtronic was building these stimulators in quantity. That supplemented their income from selling Sanborn (now Hewlett-Packard) ECG machines and from occasionally repairing TV sets, when things really got slow.

Palmer Hermundslie, a local lumber dealer, was married to Connie's sister, and he provided financial support for the early ventures and assumed responsibility for all new construction. All of the early pacemaker companies had their growth stunted by inadequate planning and lack of facilities when they were needed. Medtronic always seemed to have the buildings and the benches ready just when they were needed and rarely had to tell doctors they couldn't deliver a pacemaker. I attribute most of this superb planning to Hermundslie.

James Anderson, himself a capable design engineer, was sales manager and was always on the road in the company plane, selling something to somebody. Norman Hagfors and Robert Wingrove, both former Sunday school students of Bakken's, headed up the engineering, and Ronald Gymrek handled quality control. This was the team.

In early 1961, James Anderson and Palmer Hermundslie (both

pilots), flew in to Buffalo from Minneapolis. At a luncheon table in the Airways Hotel at the Buffalo Airport, we worked out a license agreement. The next day we had it notarized at a local bank. I don't know that the agreement was ever formalized into legal language, but it was the beginning of the Medtronic Chardack-Greatbatch implantable cardiac pacemaker, which dominated the field for the next decade.

The license agreement was a very tight one. I assumed design control for all Medtronic implantable pacemakers. I signed every drawing, every change, and had to approve every procurement source. The device had to be called a "Chardack-Greatbatch implantable cardiac pacemaker" in all company brochures, advertising, and communications, both within the company and without. Quality control reported directly to me for ten years. I sat on the board of directors. I had major (and noisy) input into all company affairs, selling pacemakers, and particularly on the dropping of unprofitable product lines like cardiac monitors and AC defibrillators. Medtronic had been in a precarious financial situation in 1960, but substantially recovered within two years and became number one in pacemakers. Today, in 2000, Medtronic is still number one.

I made monthly trips to Minneapolis to monitor the production line, to go over quality control records with Gymrek, to sign off drawings and changes, and to attend board meetings. Dr. William Chardack was just as active as I, but in an unofficial, behind-the-scenes stance. His papers, his case reports, his spring-coil electrodes, and his personal recommendations really "sold" the Medtronic device to the profession. His professional stature and reputation in the field were unparalleled. I still say he was Medtronic's most effective and most credible salesman.

We soon found that the highest grade military components were not good enough for the "zero defect" requirements of pacemakers. The warm moist environment of the human body proved a far more hostile environment than outer space or the bottom of the sea. We had predicted a five year pacemaker in our first 1959 paper.[6] But by 1970, we were only getting two years.

We spent most of the decade expanding the quality control programs. These included 100 percent testing and traceability of component lots. We instituted a thirty-day heat/mechanical shock cycle on transistors, and a 100 percent X-ray analysis of batteries and completed pacemakers. These procedures are more completely described in chapters 2 and 4.

The miniature United Transformer Company (UTC) DOT-1 transformers were wound with exceptionally fine wire and proved troublesome. UTC made a special high-reliability model with a double encasement, but we still experienced failures until we finally went to a transformerless design. The Medtronic 5862 (my last design for Medtronic) used a three-transistor, transformerless, complementary multivibrator circuit (after Roger Russell's patent) which could not "hang up" (go into paralysis after a heavy shock as from defibrillation of the patient). With diode-isolated dual battery packs and voltage-doubler output, it was probably the most reliable of the mercury-powered pacemakers of the 1960s. I was so intent on achieving rate stability that I didn't even include an end-of-life indicator in the design. Some of these units lasted almost five years, after which time they had to be electively removed because there was no way of knowing how much battery life was left.

Our epoxy encapsulant contracted when the epoxy cured, putting pressure on diodes and capacitors and sometimes crushing them. This was solved by covering each component with a protective silicone rubber sheath, by dipping it into silicone medical adhesive thinned with heptane. Tantalum capacitors failed occasionally. We finally replaced individual capacitors with banks of four series paralleled capacitors so that at least two simultaneous capacitor failures would be needed to incapacitate a pulse generator. Embarrassingly enough, with the additional exposure of the three extra capacitors, the reliability proved worse.

THE WAY IT WAS

Many of the early Medtronic programs were first worked out in Clarence, New York, and then taken to Minneapolis. I had two ovens set up in my bedroom. My wife did much of the testing. The shock test consisted of striking the transistor with a wooden pencil while measuring beta (current gain). We found that a metal pencil could wreck the transistor, but a wooden pencil could not. Many mornings I would awake to the cadence of my wife Eleanor tap, tap, tapping the transistors with her calibrated pencil. For some months every transistor that was used worldwide in Medtronic pacemakers got tapped in my bedroom.

Early transistors were inconsistent. We identified several failure modes due to contamination and leaky seals. We adopted the policy of segregating the transistors into beta classes and then heat-soaking them for five hundred hours at 125°C with five cycles of dry ice during this period. Any transistor that developed leakage or drifted more than one beta class was discarded. This was followed by a shock test. We lost about 15 percent of some of the transistors in this program, but we never lost one subsequently in a pacemaker. It is interesting to note that the "Minuteman" space program for high-reliability missile components later adopted much the same program after we had published our procedures.

LATER MEDTRONIC YEARS

We gradually worked our reliability up to the point where the battery quality became our limiting factor. It became increasingly apparent that we would never achieve our objective of a "lifetime pacemaker" with the zinc-mercury battery. I pressured Bakken to set up his own battery facility since I felt sure his suppliers would never do what needed to be done. He finally took my advice, but not until over five years later. In the meantime I again felt led to reverse careers. I terminated my license with Medtronic (under friendly circumstances) and became a battery manufacturer, which I knew nothing about.

We looked into nuclear batteries, rechargeable batteries, biological batteries, and other chemical battery systems. Our work with these systems is detailed in chapter 4, but it suffices to say here that (1) we discarded biological batteries because of their low energy density and their inconsistent performance; (2) we discarded rechargeable batteries because the battery life, with recharging, was less than the battery life of our primary batteries, without recharging; and (3) we put an intensive two-year effort into atomic batteries but finally discarded them because of the unacceptability in the clinical situation of the restrictive regulatory requirements on patient mobility and physician reporting.

In 1970–72 we finally settled on a battery with a lithium anode; an iodine cathode; and a solid-state, self-healing crystalline electrolyte. This eventually removed the battery as the limiting factor in pacemaker longevity. Today nearly every pacemaker uses a lithium battery of some sort, and nearly every surgical intervention for a pacemaker problem is electrode-related rather than battery-related.

THE ADVENT OF DEMAND PACING

In 1964, Dr. Barough Berkovitz (also an early member of our Buffalo Medical Electronics PGME chapter, when the American Optical Company medical electronic division was in Buffalo) published a series of papers on a new pacemaker concept in which the pacemaker "listened" to the heart and worked only when the heart didn't. The pacemaker worked only "on demand" and came to be known as a demand pacemaker. This seemed like quite a good idea and we ourselves began working on an implantable version. My laboratory notebook says that we completed our first successful breadboard on January 20, 1965. This design went on to become the Medtronic Model 5841 (U.S. Patent 3, 478, 746) which was the first implantable inhibited demand pacemaker (VVI) to become commercially available.

A TRIBUTE

These were times of considerable stress. We were still working out our designs and procedures and Dr. Chardack and I were not always in agreement on what should be done. At times we had some pretty harsh words. Time has mellowed all that and now I can more fully appreciate all he did. In my opinion Dr. Chardack was the epitome of all a doctor should be. He was an excellent surgeon, physician, and chemist. His concern for his patients was legendary. Many times he sat up all night at a patient's bedside, titrating in one drug, watching the response, cancelling it out, and titrating in another. Many a patient is alive today because of both his formal and his intuitive knowledge of drugs and blood chemistry and his unwavering commitment to see a patient through. When we lost a patient, I have seen him go into actual physical shock while we went over all the details of the case to see if we might have erred somewhere. I have known many dedicated doctors in my work, but few with his breadth of knowledge and his intense commitment to the professional ethic.

The design was unique in that it used a grounded-base input transistor with a very low input impedance of 5,000 ohms. My feeling was that we should match the impedance of the heart to get the best possible QRS input signal (generated by the heart), so I used a grounded-base transistor for the input stage. It was a successful design that stayed on the market for some years, but was "engineering heresy" (Dr. Peter Patton's term; he's a Minneapolis pacemaker consultant) in that conventional wisdom would tend toward high input impedance rather than low. In fact, all pacemaker designs since then have used high input impedances, in the megohms. I'm not sure the change was a good one.

Another unique feature was the lack of any built-in refractory period (the time between the QRS heartbeat wave and the "T" recovery wave during which the heart will not respond to stimulus). The high surface capacity of the platinum electrode provided an electrochemical refractory that was quite effective, if imprecise.

The circuit was the ultimate in simplicity, with only six transistors. It was always our practice to get the most we could out of the fewest number of parts. Richard Frazier, one of the "old-timers" at CAL, always said, "The best way to keep a part from failing is not to put it in in the first place!" I guess that philosophy has gone by the board now with very large scale integration (VLSI). Modern pacemaker designers think nothing of putting a million transistors into a design.

CONCLUSION

The first half-decade of pacemaking culminated in a "gathering of the clan" at several meetings in the mid-1960s. We held a symposium here in Buffalo in 1965. Three meetings sponsored by the New York Academy of Sciences similarly drew worldwide participation. William Glenn organized a pacemaker meeting in 1964, Walter Feder a meeting on bioelectrodes in 1968, and Seymour Furman a pacemaker meeting in 1969. These four meetings, among others, established pacemaking as a universally accepted procedure and cleared the way for rapid progress, both in the technical level of the apparatus and in the spreading of the word to general practitioners. Hans Lagergren, in a paper,[7] reviewed the accomplishments of the Swedish Karolinska group and recalled our Buffalo meeting where he was able to present the cases of 305 pacemaker patients from five European clinics. He expressed fear that people would forget the things that the pioneers had done.

No, Hans, many of us remember and we will never forget.

NOTES

1. W. Greatbatch et al., "A Transistorized Implantable Pacemaker for the Long Term Correction of Complete Atrio-ventricular Block." *Proc. New England Res. and Engin. Meeting* (New England Regional Engineering Meeting [NEREM]), Boston 1 (1959): 8.

2. H. Lagergren, "How It Happened: My Recollection of Early Pacing." *Pacing and Clinical Electrophysiology (PACE)* 1 (1978): 140.

3. W. Chardack et al., "A Transistorized, Self-contained, Implantable Pacemaker for the Long-term Correction of Complete Heart Block." *Surgery* 48, no. 4 (1960): 643.

4. A. Senning, "Problems with Pacemakers." *Journal of Cardiovascular Surgery* (1964).

5. S. Furman et al., "An Intracardiac Pacemaker for Stokes-Adams Seizures." *New Eng. J. Med.* 261 (1959): 943.

6. W. Greatbatch et al., "A Transistorized Implantable Pacemaker for the Long Term Correction of Complete Atrio-ventricular Block," 8.

7. Lagergren, "How It Happened," 140.

FOR FURTHER READING

Greatbatch, W., *Fifty Years of Engineering.* BENT (journal of Tau Beta Pi), 2000.

2

PULSE GENERATOR DESIGN

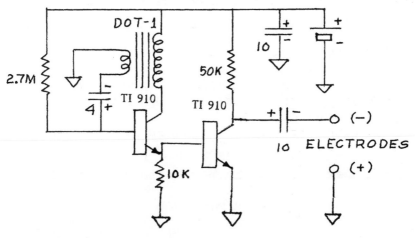

Epoxy Encapsulated Pulse Generators

The first pacemaker was implanted by our group in an experimental animal on May 7, 1958.

We were so naive as to believe that the pacemaker could be sealed against the body environment by simply wrapping it in electrical tape. It actually worked for about four hours in a dog before body fluid infiltrated the tape and shorted it out.

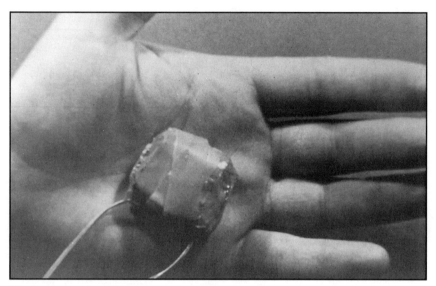

The first pacemaker, 1958.

It soon became clear that any void in any nonhermetically sealed device in the body would eventually fill with fluid.

Since we could not hermetically seal our devices (because of the hydrogen gas evolution from the mercury battery), we chose to eliminate voids and potted the circuit and battery solidly in epoxy. We also soon learned not to use insulation board and not to use insulated wire. Epoxy

THE WAY IT WAS

Within three weeks of the day that Dr. Chardack expressed interest in an implantable pacemaker I had assembled a model and brought it to the animal lab at the Buffalo, New York Veterans Hospital. Dr. Chardack and Dr. Andrew Gage (later chief of staff there) exposed the heart of a dog, and we touched the wires to the dog's heart. The heart proceeded to beat in synchrony with the device. Dr. Chardack looked at the oscilloscope, looked back at the animal, and said, "Well, I'll be damned." I quote from page 90 of my laboratory notebook number 2, written in 1959: "I seriously doubt if anything I ever do will ever give me the elation I felt that day when my own two-cubic-inch piece of electronic design controlled a living heart."

THE WAY IT WAS

We prepared an experimental animal in such a way as to demonstrate live, for a local seminar, the effect of a Stokes-Adam attack. We built a special pacemaker with a stainless steel diaphragm on the side with an air pocket and a microswitch behind it. By pressing on the diaphragm from outside the animal, we could activate the microswitch, disable the pacemaker, and put the animal into syncope (cardiac arrest). It worked fine for a day or two, but then all the air diffused out through the silicone sheath and the resulting pressure left the switch permanently activated and the animal in block. Every time we wanted to demonstrate the animal, we had to first inject a little air into the microswitch compartment with a hypodermic needle.

would not bond to either. We wired the components with solid bare wire and left our circuit mechanically floating on the wires. The epoxy completely isolated each component from its neighbor and contracted onto the wire upon curing, forming a compression bond that would allow neither water molecules nor salt ions to migrate along the wire.

We found that gas (including water vapor) would readily diffuse through both the epoxy and the silicone sheath around it, raising the interior to an eventual 100 percent humidity. Thus our electronics were essentially operating under distilled water. After all, the anodes of powerful radio transmitting tubes operate at thousands of volts with distilled cooling water in direct contact with the anodes. This is safe, but should a pinch of salt get into the cooling system, the transmitter will go through the roof! This meant that we had to keep all salt ions out. A fingerprint on a transistor anode lead would leave enough salt to create anodic corrosion, which after a time left only a residue of black powder oxide in place of the stainless steel anode wire lead. This could mean failed pacemakers.

Our original encapsulation technique involved potting the floating circuit (no printed-circuit board or other laminated mounting means) in an epoxy block in three steps. In the first step only enough epoxy was added to glue all the electronic component parts together, side by side, while their ends were externally held in a fixed position. The potted assembly looked like a pile of firewood and came to be known as "cordwood" construction. Next the circuit was hand-soldered and further cast into a monolithic starlike structure, shaped to fit in the interstices of the battery pack. The module was then inserted into the battery pack and the whole assembly potted a third time. We tried to leave at least 2mm of epoxy around the sides, top, and bottom. The device was cured overnight at 37°C and removed from the mold. Finally, a thin bonding coat of Dow Corning medical adhesive was applied. This was finger-applied to the cured pulse generator and then a final coat of white Dow Corning RTV 502 was poured over the top and allowed to drip down the sides. After two hours of curing, the pulse generator was turned over, trimmed flush with a scalpel, and more RTV 502 was poured on to complete the covering. We studied various silicone coatings. We would have preferred a one-part, heat-cure mix since it contained fewer additives, but our pulse generator would not withstand the temperature of the cure cycle. We looked at RTV 501 (a tan-colored silicone) which handled a little better than RTV 502, but which had mercury in its accelerator. We settled on the RTV 502 after deciding that its tin accelerator was safer. Many such judgments were guesses made quickly because there just wasn't much data around on the long-term behavior of materials in the body.

The first units were serialized by shaping pieces of bare wire into numbers and dropping them on the uncured silicone. The wires were removed after cure, leaving a depressed hardened meniscus identification number. Later production units had the Medtronic company name and the Chardack-Greatbatch identification machined into the final aluminum mold. The serial number was punched out on a plastic tape and changed for each pouring.

THE WAY IT WAS

After implantation, a very tight collagenous sheath grew around the pulse generator, closely conforming to every indentation. When such a pulse generator was removed, the Chardack-Greatbatch lettering remained imprinted, backward, in the collagen sheath in the patient. We felt this was really leaving our mark.

Pulse Generator Nomenclature

Implantable pulse generators have progressed from the simple two-transistor, fixed-rate stimulators, which I first described forty years ago, to the extremely complicated multichamber, programmable devices of the

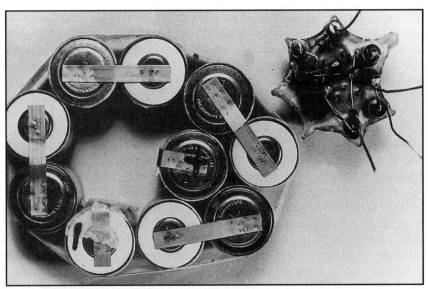

Epoxy cordwood module, ready for assembly into battery.

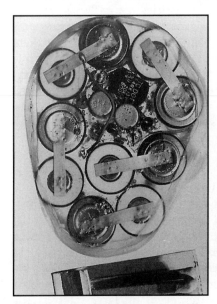

Epoxy potted assembly ready for attachment of silicone sheath and leads.

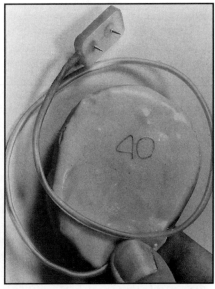

Our first clinically implanted pacemaker, April 15, 1960. Note that electrode leads are permanently attached: no connectors.

present. After the first decade, it became clear that a standard nomenclature was needed to precisely identify the type of pulse generator one was talking about. Dr. Victor Parsonnet et al. introduced a first system using a three-digit symbol to describe the pacemaker's function.[1] The first digit identified the driven chamber, the second digit identified the sensed chamber, if any, and the third digit identified the mode of operation of the demand function, if any. The earliest fixed-rate pacemakers, mentioned above, stimulated the ventricle but had no sensing function. Thus they were termed VOO. The first external "demand" pacemaker of Dr. Barough Berkowitz[2] and the similar implantable devices of mine[3] stimulated the ventricle. But if they sensed a QRS (stimulating impulse) wave on the ventricle, they inhibited the pacemaker function. Thus they worked only "on demand" and were termed "demand pacemakers," and were thus termed VVI. Subsequent demand pacemakers of Walter Keller[4] asynchronously fired a stimulus into the ventricle if no QRS was sensed, but directly into the QRS if triggered by one. If a QRS was sensed, the pacemaker fired into the ventricle during the QRS. Since this was during the refractory period, no stimulation resulted. Thus Keller's device was a demand pacemaker which fired noneffective impulse into a beating heart. Thus it was termed VVT. Table 1 classifies the early pacemakers using this method.

The advent of multichamber and multiprogrammable pacemakers during the third decade of pacing necessitated a more detailed terminology, although unfortunately it was created at the expense of simplicity. Parsonnet et al.[5] again rose to the challenge with an expanded nomenclature. Table 2 shows the classification of the more complex pacemaker systems using Parsonnet's newer expanded terminology.

Fixed Rate Pacemakers

The first implantable pacemakers simply fired a 2 millisecond (ms) electrical pulse into the heart. Most early pulse generators used four, five, or six 1.35v (volt) mercury cell batteries (except for our first 10-cell monsters) so that the unloaded open-circuit voltage (OCV) output of the pacemaker was about 5 to 8 volts in amplitude. This was several times threshold (the minimally required stimulating impulse) for many early electrodes. However, the uncertainty of performance of these early structures was such that often even this large safety factor was not always enough. But the objective was simply to drive the heart, without much regard for economy of battery life, competition (between the heart and the pacemaker), or synchrony of the cardiac chambers. These early devices accomplished their purpose, even

TABLE 1
SUGGESTED NOMENCLATURE CODE FOR IMPLANTABLE CARDIAC PACEMAKERS

Chamber paced	Chamber sensed	Mode of response	Generic description	Previously used designation
V	0	0	Ventricular pacing; no sensing function	Asynchronous; fixed rate; set rate
A	0	0	Atrial pacing; no sensing function	Atrial fixed rate; atrial asynchronous
D	0	0	Atrioventricular pacing; no sensing function	AV sequential fixed rate (asynchronous)
V	V	I	Ventricular pacing and sensing, inhibited mode	Ventricular inhibited; R inhibited; R blocking; R suppressed; noncompetitive inhibited; demand; standby
V	V	T	Ventricular pacing and sensing, triggered mode	Ventricular triggered; R triggered; R wave stimulated; noncompetitive triggered; following; R synchronous; demand; standby
A	A	I	Atrial pacing and sensing, inhibited mode	Atrial inhibited; P inhibited; P blocking; P suppressed
A	A	T	Atrial pacing and sensing, triggered mode	Atrial triggered; P triggered; P stimulated; P synchronous
V	A	T	Ventricular pacing, atrial sensing, triggered mode	Atrial synchronous, atrial synchronized, AV synchronous
D	V	I	Atrioventricular pacing, ventricular sensing, inhibited mode	Bifocal sequential demand, AV sequential

From V. Parsonnet et al., *Circulation* 50, 1974.

TABLE 2
FIVE POSITION PACEMAKER CODE
I C H D

Position	I	II	III	IV	V
Category	Chamber(s) paced	Chamber(s) sensed	Mode of response	Programmable functions	Special tachyarrhythmia functions
Letters Used	V- Ventricle	V- Ventricle	T-Triggered	P-Program-mable (rate and/ or output)	B-Bursts
	A- Atrium	A- Atrium	I-Inhibited	M-Multi-programmable	N-Normal Rate Competition
	D- Double	D- Double	D-Double* O-None		S-Scanning
		O-None	R-Reverse	O-None	E-External
Manu-facturer's Designation Only	S- Single Chamber	S- Single Chamber			
			Comma optional here		

*Atrial triggered and ventricular inhibited.

From V. Parsonnet et al., *PACE* 4, no. 4, 1981.

though the batteries, the electrodes, and even the electronic components themselves often left much to be desired.

When the first five years of successful pacing had been achieved, investigators began seeking ways to make the pacemaker more "physiological." We had never been as enthusiastic as some about this objective. We were probably too pure in our engineering approach, but we saw Mother Nature as one of the greatest killers of all times. We didn't like to see her assisted in this morbid endeavor by giving a life-saving device a controlling input. That input may be provided by some well understood variables, but it may well be subject to some that are not so well known. Goldreyer points out that "physiological pacing" is a philosophical term that has different meanings to different people.[6] Atrioventricular (AV) synchrony is not equatable to physiologic pacing. He states that increasing the rate, in synchrony, can be most inappropriate if reentry mechanisms cause simultaneous filling of atria and ventricles. If the patient has neural feedback such that both the atrium and ventricle fill at the same time, speeding up the heart rate with a demand pacemaker could be dangerous. Cardiac output can drop dramatically to dangerous levels. Nevertheless, the trend has been towards controlling the pacemaker rate and function, to cause it to depart from its comfortable one-per-second, lifetime rhythm.

The Function of Non-fixed-rate Pacemakers

Many patients have near-normal heart function most of the time and only occasionally go into cardiac arrest. In these patients, the fixed-rate pacemaker competes against their own physiological pacemaker (natural heart rhythm) much of the time. Worse yet, as the stimulation pulse drifts through the ECG waveform, a stimulation pulse will eventually inevitably fall into the "T" wave, into what is known as the "vulnerable period." In the presence of a hyperexcitable myocardium, as would exist in the presence of a new infarct, such a stimulation pulse in the vulnerable period could well elicit a run of tachycardia or even fibrillation.

DEMAND PACEMAKERS

In the mid-1960s, my good friend Barough Berkovitz conceived an external pacemaker design that would function only when the heart did not.[7] It operated only on demand and came to be known as a demand pacemaker. It consisted of both an ECG amplifier and a conventional pacemaker stimulator with circuitry added to cause an output from the ECG amplifier to inhibit the stimulator. Thus its ECHD classification was VVI. We were impressed by Berkovitz's work and began developing an implantable version. We were still using our two-transistor blocking oscillator and added a four-transistor QRS amplifier to it. My patent notebook shows this circuit first reduced to practice on February 17, 1965.

This circuit finally matured into the Medtronic Model 5841 pacemaker in 1966.[8] It was the first commercially available implantable VVI pacemaker and remained a popular device for some years.

Subsequently, Walter Keller adapted his P-wave pacemaker to be responsive to ventricular activity.[9] However, Keller triggered his pacemaker to fire innocuously into the R wave of a sensed heartbeat, so this ECHD classification was VVT. The VVT pacemaker presented some advantages. Pacemaker function was immediately apparent as a spike in the R wave of the ECG, whereas a failed VVI pacemaker could not be detected during normal heart rhythm. (Later VVI designs incorporated a reed switch activated by a hand-held magnet to convert the pulse generator to VOO at a free-running "magnet rate" for testing.) Also, the VVT pacemaker would continue to pace, albeit at a somewhat higher rate, in

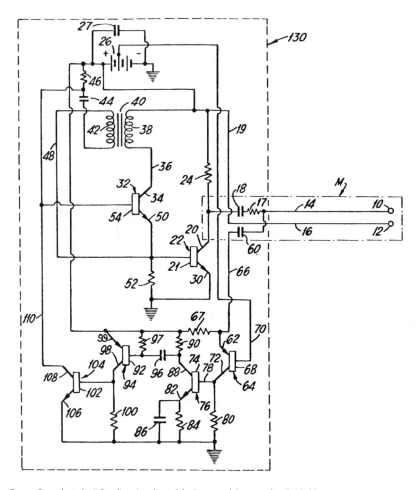

From Greatbatch, "Cardiac Implantable Demand Pacemaker," 1965.

the presence of heavy electromagnetic or myoelectric interference, which would inhibit a VVI pacemaker, the reason people with pacemakers were told to stay away from microwave ovens.

Interference Signals

The inhibitory effect of myoelectric signals from the pectoral muscles has become a matter of increasing concern to many physicians. It is a major problem with unipolar electrodes. The "antenna length" of a unipolar system, i.e., the distance between the electrode tip and the metal case of the pulse generator, may be 20cm or more, while in a bipolar system, it is only the distance between the tip and the ring on the catheter, which is about 2cm. Thus, unipolar pacemakers are an order of magnitude more sensitive to myoelectric interference than are bipolar systems. The situation was critical enough for Dr. Seymour Furman to organize a symposium of papers in which he said "the incidence of inhibition may be one-third of all unipolar pacemakers implanted."[10] In the symposium, Dr. Robert Hauser declared it "a major clinical problem" and stated that the bipolar electrode system was much to be preferred for multiprogrammable, multichamber pacemakers. However, bipolar electrode systems are structurally larger and more difficult to build. Thus most manufacturers are still introducing unipolar systems in multichamber pacemakers. This subject is treated in more detail in a subsequent chapter on electrodes.

Furman notes that "one manufacturer" seemed much more free of myoelectric interference. Subsequently Lawrence Shearon reported that Medtronic uses a "signal averaging" technique to discriminate against 50/60 Hz and myoelectric activity.[11]

The major disadvantage of the VVT pacemaker was its high current consumption. Inhibited VVI pulse generators consume only a small fraction of the battery current required for continual pulsing. The VVT pacemaker remains at high current drain, pulsing the heart, whether needed or not. Thus, theoretically at least, batteries should last considerably longer in a VVI design. It is this factor that has caused the VVT pacemaker to fade from popularity in recent years.

All of the above devices were cast into epoxy blocks. It was not feasible to attempt to hermetically seal these devices as long as the power supply was a mercury battery. Some investigators did try, but it was necessary to go to engineering extremes, and truly successful designs were not achieved before a new development foretold the end of the mercury pacemaker battery. That was the hermetically sealed lithium battery.

In our early work on demand pacemakers we did considerable work trying to characterize the frequency spectrum of a physiological QRS wave, as did others. Some used a half-sine wave and others used a square pulse. We tried many stimulator waveforms and eventually settled on a single sine wave at 30 Hz, starting at about 240° in the cycle and continuing for another 360.°

We found the following waveform to be very close to the spectrum of a normal QRS. An important feature was that it was precisely mathematically describable and hence precisely repeatable, being easily generated from commercially available function generators. Thus a 2 mv QRS wave, meeting this specification, would be the same on anyone's test equipment, anywhere in the world. Unfortunately, no one else shared my views and we were the only ones to ever use it. I still think it is a good waveform.

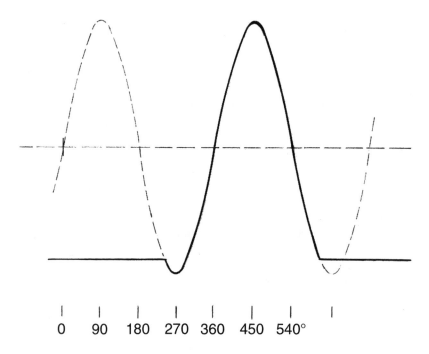

0   90   180   270   360   450   540°

A modified sine wave.

The Relative Merits of Demand and Fixed-Rate Pacemakers

The fixed-rate VOO pacemaker, once the only type available, has now declined in usage to an insignificant level. We question the wisdom of such a complete abandonment.

Chardack, after extended animal trials, suggested that there was little hazard from competition in a heart with no infarct or with a mature infarct.[12] After having allowed innumerable high-energy pacemaker impulses to drift through the ECG waveform, he stated that it was not the pacemaker impulse at all that initiated a fibrillation. Rather, it was the action potential that was initiated by the pacemaker impulse which propagated across the heart and caused fibrillation if it passed a hyperexcitable area, such as a new infarct. Thus a heart at risk from competition would probably shortly electrocute itself on one of its own extrasystoles anyway.

It is comforting to know I am not completely alone in my opinion. Paul Zoll, William Chardack, and Adrian Kantrowitz have all expressed similar views. At least I'm in very good company.

The medical literature nowhere (as of 1983) proves a clear-cut decrease in risk in a large population with demand pacemakers. Several large studies demonstrate no significant increase in longevity for patients with demand pacemakers as against those with fixed-rate pacemakers. Furman stated that the fixed-rate pacemaker solved the problem of bradycardia.[13] Although there may be a clear-cut improvement in the quality of life, there is, in our admittedly biased opinion, no demonstrable increase in longevity with the more complex devices.

We believe that all temporary pacemakers should be of the demand type and we would be the last to suggest that all implantable pacemakers should be VOO, but we think they are perfectly adequate for extending the lives of a much larger population than now receive them.

We bring up this point because in 2000, MRI (magnetic resonance imaging) is generally contraindicated for pacemaker patients. What is needed is an MRI-proof pacemaker. We suspect such a device will prove difficult to build in other than a VOO configuration, due to the intense MRI magnetic field which could well incapacitate, or even destroy, a conventional pacemaker.

It may well prove desirable, if a pacemaker patient truly needs repetitive MRI procedures, to replace the conventional pacemaker with an MRI-proof VOO pacemaker. Particularly in the case of a patient in complete block, one who has presented at least once with Stokes-Adam syndrome (a fainting attack), the physician might decide to leave the MRI-proof VOO pacemaker permanently installed, in view of the above considerations.

Nonatrial Rate Responsive Pacemaking Systems*

Donaldson et al. reported fifteen patients treated with a Vitatron TX1 rate-responsive QT pacemaker, whose rate varied with the averaged QT interval.[14] The pacemaker is programmed by means of a radio frequency telemetry link to an external HP85 computer. Donaldson suggests this as a substitute for atrial synchronous pacing, particularly in patients with atrial dysfunction.

K. Anderson described a new pacemaker design that is rate-responsive to integrated muscle activity, increasing its rate during exercise.[15] He provided a 10 second attack integral and a forty-eight second decay integral in signal averaging. Camilli in Italy demonstrated considerable clinical experience with a pacemaker system that sensed the pH of the blood and varied pacing rate accordingly.[16] Both Funke[17] and Krassner[18] reported pacing systems which regulated heart rate from respiration rate.

---

*Much more modern references are available supplementing these 1980s examples.

Lastly, Wirtzfeld reported a pacemaker system that measured the oxygen saturation of the blood and varied the heart rate accordingly.[19]

All of these developments demonstrate the desire of many investigators to arrive at rate-responsive systems, but without having to assume the difficult and uncertain task of sensing and driving in the atrium.

Other Pacing Modalities

H. Anderson in Denmark reported thirteen patients paced by means of a noninvasive balloon esophageal electrode having three redundant indifferent electrodes.[20] He used a 12ms pulse and reported thresholds of 2 to 10mA (5mA avg.) at 16 to 25v. He stated that pacing at over 15mA produced pain and/or discomfort. He can pace either the ventricle or the auricle, depending on the positioning of the electrode. This is a revival of a very old technique first taught by Shafiroff[21] and by Burack and Furman.[22] We have thought such an approach to be attractive but physicians to whom we have talked tend to discourage it, due to the difficulty of placing the electrode, and the danger of a gag reflex on a critical cardiac patient. Most cardiologists seem to feel that the passing of a conventional temporary transvenous catheter is a preferred procedure.

Transformerless Pacemakers

Up until the mid-1960s we were still using pretty much the original two-transistor, transformer-coupled blocking oscillator. As we overcame problems in other components, the transformer and the battery began to stand out as principal causes of pulse generator failure. We tried many multivibrator circuits in an attempt to eliminate the transformer, but each had some bad feature. Some were unstable against varying battery voltage. Others were temperature sensitive. A surprising number, some of which were in rather high-volume pacemaker production, were not self-starting. They could "hang up" under certain conditions and not function at all. We finally settled on a highway flasher circuit that had been invented by one of our people, Roger Russell (U.S. Patent 3,508,167). This was a unique three-transistor circuit which could not hang up and whose rate was relatively insensitive to changes in battery voltage. We combined this with a voltage doubler of my own design (U.S. Patent 4,050,004), which was a takeoff on some of the very high voltage lightning machines I had seen at Cornell. It was unique in that its grounded output could be connected to one side of the battery. All other doublers we had seen necessitated floating the battery, a distinct disadvantage if you wanted to incorporate a "demand" ECG amplifier operating against ground. The combi-

THE WAY IT WAS

I provided three outputs: a singler, a doubler, and a tripler, providing 2.7v, 5.5v, and 8v OCV on three separate stainless steel posts. Each post was drilled so that a Siemens-type electrode lead could pass through all three. A pointed stainless steel set screw was inserted in one of the three posts and forced down until the point pierced the polyethylene insulation, connecting the lead to the desired output. The output could thus be raised or lowered to the next higher or lower level by simply moving the set screw to another post. I thought it was a great idea, but (the story of my life!) no one else did, and it was never used. I still keep some of the posts to demonstrate my eternal optimism!

nation matured into the Medtronic (VOO) Model 5862 pacemaker, which was the last circuit I designed for them.

A decade later, I built this same circuit with a lithium battery into a tripler circuit that provided an open-circuit voltage (OCV) of over eight volts from a 2.8v cell.

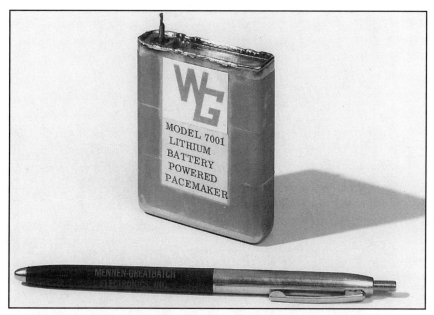

First lithium pacemaker prototype, 1970. (Inept weld made by the author!)

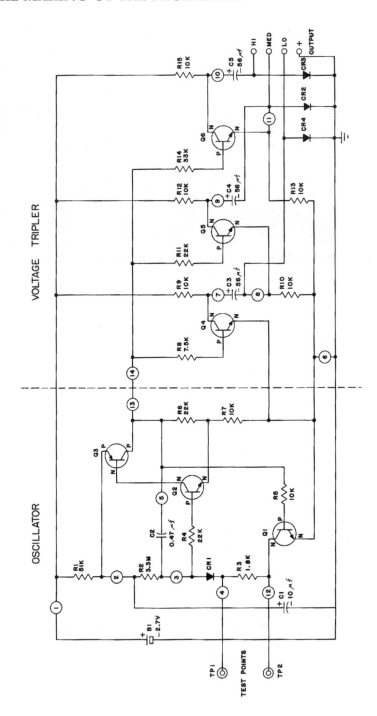

Transformerless pacemaker circuit with tripler output.

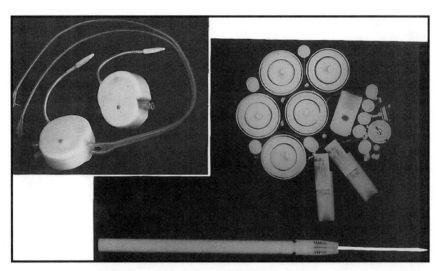

1974 Programmable Pacemaker, with "Programmer" (x-ray view on right). Note that the batteries are completely discharged.

LITHIUM PACEMAKER STRUCTURE

The advent of the lithium battery had a major impact on pacemaking and on the reliability and longevity of implanted pulse generators. Furman has said that the lithium battery was the most significant pacemaker improvement since the pacemaker was invented. The lithium battery's impact on pulse generators came partly through its own superior reliability, but a major additional factor was that it made pulse generators sealable. The lack of any gas evolution meant that pulse generators could be laser-welded into a metal can with a glass-metal hermetic terminal. All the circuitry and the battery operated in a dry environment. All pacemakers are built this way today, and failures from premature battery exhaustion or moisture infiltration are rare. Further details on the lithium power source are in chapter 4.

Thus the epoxy encapsulated mercury-powered pulse generator of the 1960s gave way to the lithium-powered, metal encased, hermetically sealed device of the 1970s, 1980s, and 1990s.

PROGRAMMABLE PULSE GENERATORS

Probably the first programmable pacemaker was a General Electric design in the early 1960s described by Dr. Adrian Kantrowitz.[23] This device used a latching reed relay actuated by an external magnet. It permitted a choice of one of two fixed rates.

Another early programmable device was described by our group[24] and enabled variation of both rate and amplitude. The device required the use of a percutaneous Kieth needle. The implanted pulse generator would be palpated and the control protrusions located. The Kieth needle was then inserted percutaneously into one of the two control protrusions and rotated to control either rate or amplitude. The control protrusions consisted of a variable resistor with an attached stainless steel guide, covered by a silicone rubber sheath. A stainless steel adapter received the three-sided Kieth needle like an Allen wrench and transmitted the torque to the shaft of the variable resistor. Neoprene grommets around each moving part sealed the variable resistor against infiltration of body fluid. The silicone rubber sheath closed upon withdrawal of the Kieth needle, providing a further seal.

These controls were incorporated in Medtronic Model 5870 pacemakers for several years. However, the need for a percutaneous puncture meant that doctors rarely used them, although they seemed happy to have them available, just in case they were ever needed. We

---

THE WAY IT WAS

We made the first Kieth needle adapters out of epoxy which we cast in silicone rubber molds to approximate shape and then machined out on our old fourth-hand, forty-year-old Atlas lathe (I still have it in my shop). However, the sharp Kieth needle point tended to dig into the funnel-shaped walls of the adapter rather than sliding freely by. It was obvious that we needed stainless steel adapters but our old Atlas wouldn't handle the material and no local shop would take on the job of machining the triangular hole.

A local entrepreneur, John Nicholas, had a machine shop in which he handled small lots of very large machines (like turbine rotors from the St. Lawrence Seaway) that were too big for any of the other machines in our area. Nicholas was sympathetic to our problem and offered to help. He machined out our tiny parts on his big machine. He made the triangular hole by drilling a round hole and then swedging it around an actual Kieth needle as a onetime form. When we wanted a thousand adapters, we had to give Nicholas a thousand Kieth needles. I'm sure whatever he charged covered only a fraction of his costs. It was this kind of sympathetic cooperation from our friends that took the pacemaker from a dream to a practical device. Thank you, John!

understand that they did see some use in setting pacemaker rate and output at the time of implantation. The controls were eliminated from subsequent models.

Multichamber Programmable Pacemakers

Early atrial sensing pacemakers never achieved much more than 1 percent of the worldwide pacemaker market, mainly because they required two electrodes. Since electrodes have always given some problems, two electrodes meant double trouble. Worse yet, the early atrial electrode was an epicardial (heart surface) type which required a thoracotomy. Nevertheless, the extra 15 percent of cardiac output that was available with synchrony from a *failing* heart indicated their occasional use. One can find a number of case histories where they represented a satisfactory solution to an otherwise intractable problem.

In more recent years new atrial electrodes of the fixation or "J" types have permitted transvenous placement of electrodes in both the atrium and the ventricle without the small but significant morbidity of the thoracotomy on these elderly and poor-risk patients. These newer electrodes are detailed more completely in the subsequent chapter on the subject.

This opened the way for multichamber sensing and stimulation. The various permutations and combinations of sensing and driving in both chambers, with various delays and various logic sequences, tend to boggle the mind of this poor engineer. All these electronic possibilities combine with the physiological conductions, delays, and refractories to produce some very complex patterns. We now see some new pacemaker-induced arrhythmias that do not exist physiologically. It is possible to have retrograde physiological conduction feedback into the atrium which produces an oscillatory tachycardia which can then only be broken by a careful selection of a proper refractory time in one of the electronic circuits, with the hope that the physiological leg of the feedback circuit does not subsequently change with time.[25]

ECG analysis in the pacemaker lab (electrophysiology) has become a speciality all its own, requiring a perception and training on the part of the cardiologist that increases in complexity with each annual meeting.

IMPLANTED COMPUTER TECHNOLOGY

Contemporary pulse generators may have as many as a million transistors on a single monolithic chip no larger than a person's fingernail. Whereas early circuitry was analog in nature, most pacemaker functions

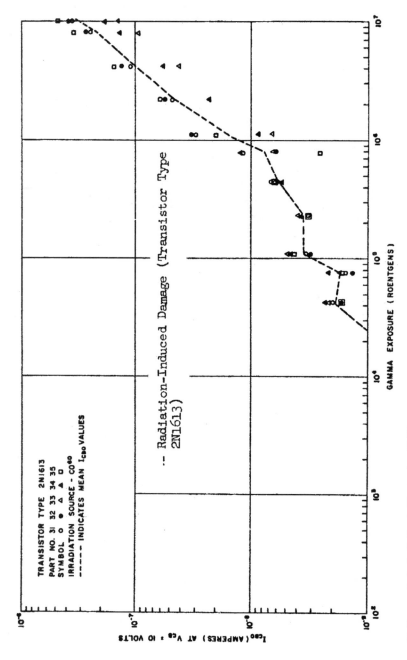

From U. Cocca et al., *Radiation in Electronics*, 1965.

such as timing, inhibiting, memory, and decision making are now performed digitally. As these functions increase in complexity it becomes more desirable to build the circuit in a rather general, computer-based architecture, with the various functions spelled out in software. Memory functions can store and summarize such things as patient name, pacemaker model, electrode type, date of implant, mode of programmed function, and even a summary of the number of times the demand function was utilized over the preceding six month period. Interrogation and control functions going in, and response and monitoring functions coming out, are accomplished by telemetry with a careful electronic validation of security to avoid accidental reprogramming by electric garage door openers and so forth.

Each pacemaker manufacturer has its own method of telemetry and validation that is quite different from every other manufacturer's system. Unfortunately, there is some overlap. One manufacturer's controller can sometimes break another manufacturer's security and perform an unwanted reprogramming which may not be immediately correctable until the proper controller is ascertained and procured. Also, the necessity for having multiple controllers creates a logistics problem. A pacemaker clinic must have a controller for each system they expect to see, perhaps as many as a dozen varieties. Unfortunately, controllers are notably subject to abuse and to system failure, and most medical centers feel that they must have one or even two backup units to be legally protected. Thus a pacemaker clinic must have twenty to forty controllers in-house and must keep all of them maintained. This is an expensive, wasteful, and totally unnecessary burden on hospital finances.

In our admittedly biased opinion, controllers and pacemakers should be compatible and interchangeable. Efforts are underway by standards committees of the Association for Advancement of Medical Instrumentation (AAMI) to implement some sort of standardization between systems. Many industries have created guidelines for a standard interface, and we see no reason why pacemaker people can't get together and do it, too.

Dr. Bernard Boal makes an impassioned plea for controller standardization.[26] R. Gold presents a manufacturer's rebuttal, which we find unconvincing.[27] Twenty years later the problem remains unsolved.

Radiation Effects on Implanted Devices

In chapter 6 on sterilization we discuss the effects of radiation on implanted devices. Since that information is pertinent here, we will present it here, as well.

Four decades ago we were involved in instrumentation for engine controls for a proposed nuclear-powered aircraft. Transistor controls, although very new at the time, were believed to be needed because of the severe vibration environment. We were, of course, greatly concerned about nuclear damage to electronic devices. Our investigation revealed that the critical component is the semiconductor and that the damage level is about 10^{13} NVT (neutrons versus time),[28] or 10^7 roentgens (measure of X-ray radiation).[29] This is far above the lethal level for humans, so we subsequently had no concern about clinical therapeutic radiation effects on pacemakers.

More recently it was discovered that therapeutic radiation was having a deleterious effect on clinically implanted pacemakers using integrated circuits. The culprit was found to be the MOSFET transistor chip. The situation was serious enough for Furman to organize a series of four papers from three countries into a symposium on the problem.[30] Pulse generator failure was clinically documented with accumulated radiation of as little as 3×10^3 rads, over three orders of magnitude less than with the older junction transistor devices. Thus it is clear that new devices need to be rechecked against the old standards.

Antiarrhythmic Pacemakers and Implantable Defibrillators

The simplest antiarrhythmic device is a VOO fixed-rate pacemaker in its normal operating function. In the face of a tachycardia or other arrhythmia, the VOO impulse will drift through the ECG waveform inevitably eventually falling into the best possible position to extinguish the arrhythmia. One wonders how many arrhythmias were automatically extinguished in the first decades of pacing by the old VOO pacemakers, without any medical attention.

Since then, a number of special pacing devices have been considered for treatment of arrhythmias. At one time "paired pulses" were tried, but the results were uncertain and unpredictable and the technique never achieved popularity. Some pacemakers have been designed to give bursts of impulses into an arrhythmia and have earned the approval of some groups.[32,33] Mirowski introduced an implantable defibrillator with a battery capacity sufficient to deliver over 100 countershocks.[34] Modern defibrillators do even better.

One must credit Dr. Mirowski for dedicated perseverance in an uphill, fifteen-year battle to convince the professions (both medical and engineering) that his device can truly save lives. The implantable cardioverter/defibrillator is now universally accepted by the medical profession.

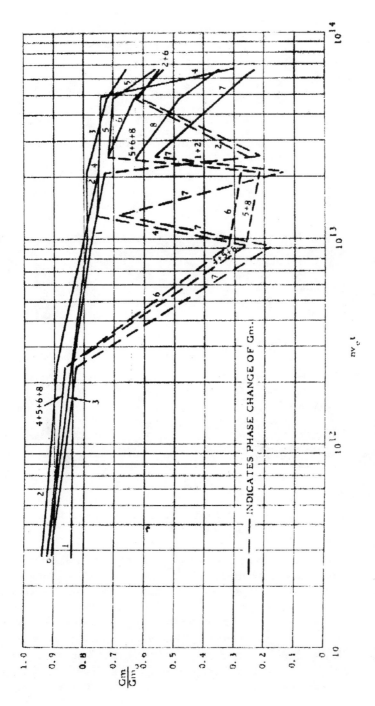

Neutron damage to semiconductors. From A. Kaufman, *Radiation Effects in Electronics*, 1965.

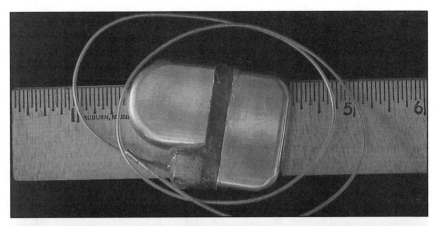

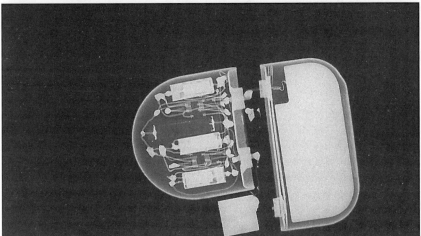

Autoclavable pacemaker pulse generator with lithium silver vanadium pentoxide battery (X-ray view below).

AUTOCLAVABLE STRUCTURES

One more area remains to be addressed. That is the sterilization of pacemaker systems. The older batteries could not withstand autoclave temperatures so older pacemakers were sterilized by other means, first by cold sterilization methods and later by ethylene oxide gas. Gas sterilizers are not available in forward areas of developing countries. Even in developed countries where they are more generally available, they must be very carefully used and very carefully maintained to be safe and effective. The overall problem of sterilization is treated in chapter 6.

Since the earlier batteries could not stand steam sterilization, pulse generator designers had few reservations about designing in components which also would not withstand these temperatures. Such components, notably Hi-K ceramic capacitors, are smaller and less expensive. Now with the availability of autoclavable batteries, autoclavable pacemakers are feasible. They could be sterilized anywhere that a home pressure cooker could be set on a charcoal stove. The next step is for pulse generator designers to redesign their circuits with 125°C tantalum capacitors and the physically larger Lo-K ceramic capacitors to enable the entire system to be autoclaved. With the batteries, it was a case of a new design, but with the components, it was a problem merely of component selection rather than component development. On the preceding page is a simple VOO pacemaker with a sealed lithium silver vanadium oxide battery and a sealed hybrid circuit that not only will withstand a thirty minute autoclave, but has operated within specifications for seven days at 130°C.

The structure in this case for a simple VOO pacemaker is two separate hermetically sealed metal cans, joined by an epoxy intermediate section. This last section contains the interconnections between the two cans and the connector. The circuit is a hybrid with transistors, diodes, and capacitors as chips on a ceramic substrate. Resistors and circuit wires are first vacuum-deposited onto the substrate. This technology permits manufacturing the complete circuits for as little as $10 each, even in quantities of as small as one hundred pieces.

We regard this structure as eminently well suited for manufacturing in underdeveloped countries. Pacemaker kits could consist of the circuit substrate, the cans, and the components. Alternatively, they could be supplied assembled, with both cans completely sealed, tested, and ready to be cast into a unit. Such a final assembly operation could be accomplished in facilities normally found in any TV repair shop, but of course under sterile conditions.

PACEMAKER COMPLEXITY—COST EFFECTIVENESS

As pacemakers have become more complex, they have become more expensive and more confusing. The diagnosis and treatment of complex arrhythmias has become literally a speciality of its own. Added to physiological arrhythmias are a few which are actually pacemaker-induced,[35] some actually life-threatening. Dr. Victor Parsonnet and others have suggested some rather strict criteria for a qualified pacemaker clinic and for pacemaker physicians.[36] Dr. Robert Hauser organized a symposium of a number of excellent papers in which recognized experts discussed these needs from a number of points of view.[37]

One sometimes wonders if the increasing complexity may not be approaching, or perhaps even a little beyond, peak cost-effectiveness. In the 1960s, we implanted a pacemaker to save a life when the indications were complete heart block with Stokes-Adam syndrome. Now a pacemaker is implanted, at much greater cost, to improve the quality of life. Thus the indications now encompass over four times as many patients as before. Parsonnet reported that the usage of pacemakers in the eastern United States exceeds one per five hundred of the general population.[38]

The fixed-rate VOO pacemaker was the lifesaver that increased the average life expectancy of a patient with the above indications from one year to that normal for a person of that age. Furman has confirmed that the VOO pacemaker solved the problem of bradycardia.[39] The more complicated pacemakers undoubtedly have their uses and may be critically needed in certain cases, but there is little evidence in the literature for any significant increase in longevity from the use of more complicated pacemakers. This is particularly true as pacemaking becomes more commonly used in developing countries. There is an economic factor to consider.

Finally, in 1983 the North American Society for Pacing and Electrostimulation adopted a position which said, "solely on the basis of patient safety, there is no indication for the implantation of a single or dual chamber pulse generator which is not programmable."[40] It is interesting to note that there were no engineers on this panel.

NOTES

1. V. Parsonnet, S. Furman, and N. Smyth, "Implantable Cardiac Pacemakers: Status Report and Resource Guideline (ICHD)." *Circulation* 50 (1974): A21.

2. B. Berkowitz, "Heart Pacing Apparatus." U.S. Patent 3,345,990, filed 1964, issued 1967.

3. W. Greatbatch, "Cardiac Implantable Demand Pacemaker." U.S. Patent 3,478,746, filed 1965, issued 1969.

4. J. W. Keller, "Standby Cardiac Pacer." U.S. Patent 3,431,912, 1966.

5. V. Parsonnet, S. Furman, and N. Smyth, "A Revised Code for Pacemaker Identification." *PACE* 4, no. 4 (1981).

6. B. Goldreyer, "Physiological Pacing: The Role of AV Synchrony." *PACE* 5, no. 4 (1982): 613.

7. Berkowitz, "Heart Pacing Apparatus."

8. Greatbatch, "Cardiac Implantable Demand Pacemaker."

9. Keller, "Standby Cardiac Pacer."

10. S. Furman, "Electromagnetic Interference." *PACE* 5, no. 1 (1982a): 1.

11. L. Shearon, "Letter to the Editor." *PACE* 6, no. 136 (1983).

12. W. Chardack, Personal communication, 1967.

13. S. Furman, "Pacemaker Programmability." *PACE* 6, no. 6 (1983): 1221.

14. R. Donaldson and A. Rickards, "Rate Responsive Pacing Using the Evoked QT Principle." *PACE* 6, no. 16 (1983): 1344.

15. K. Anderson, D. Brumwell, and S. Huntley, "A Pacemaker Which Automatically Increases Its Rate with Physical Activity." *PACE* 6, no. 3, II (1983): A12.

16. L. Camilli, "A New Pacemaker Autoregulating the Rate of Pacing in Relation to Metabolic Needs." *5th Intl. Symp. Excerpta Medica*, Amsterdam (1977): 414.

17. H. Funke, "Einn Herzschrittmacher mit belastungsabhan giger Frequenzregulation." *Biomen Technik* 20 (1975): 225.

18. J. Krasner, "A Physiologically Controlled Pacemaker." *JAAMS* 1, no. 3 (1966): 476.

19. A. Wirtzfeld, "Central Venous Oxygen Saturation for the Control of Automatic Rate-responsive Pacing." *PACE* 5 (1982): 829.

20. H. Anderson and P. Pless, "Trans-esophageal Pacing." *PACE* 6, no. 4 (1983): 674.

21. B. Shafiroff and J. Lindner, "Effects of External Electrical Pacemaker Stimuli on the Human Heart." *J. Thor. Surg.* 33 (1957): 544.

22. B. Burack and S. Furman, "Transesophagael Pacing." *J. Thor. Surg.* 33 (1957): 544.

23. A. Kantrowitz, R. Cohen, H. Raillard, J. Schmidt, and D. Feldman, "The Treatment of Complete Heart Block with an Implanted Controllable Pacemaker." *Surg. Gyn. Obstet.* 115 (1962): 415.

24. W. Chardack, A. Gage, A. Federico, G. Schimert, and W. Greatbatch, "Clinical Experience with an Implantable Pacemaker." *Annals NY Acad. Sciences* 111, no. 3 (1964): 1075.

25. R. Luderitz, N. d'Alnoncourt, G. Steinbeck, and J. Beyer, "Therapeutic Pacing in Tachyarrythmias By Implanted Pacemakers." *PACE* 5, no. 3 (1982): 366.

26. B. Boal, "Emergency Reprogramming of Cardiac Pacemakers." *PACE* 6, no. 3 (1983): 651.

27. R. Gold, S. Saulson, and D. MacGregor, "Programmable Pacing Systems: The Medium and the Message." *PACE* 5, no. 5 (1983): 776.

28. A. Kaufman, "Neutron and Neutron Spectra Contribution to Damage in Silicon Field-effect Transistors." In *Radiation Effects in Electronics,* American Society of Testing Materials (ASTM) STP 384 (1965): 60.

29. U. Cocca and N. Koepp-Baker, "Radiation Induced Surface Effects on Selected Semiconductor Devices." In *Radiation in Electronics* ASTM STP 384 (1965): 170.

30. S. Furman, "Radiation Effects on Implanted Pacemakers." *PACE* 5, no. 2 (1982b): 145.

31. J. Fischer, R. Meira, and S. Furman, "Termination of Ventricular Tachycardia with Bursts of Rapid Ventricular Pacing." *American Journal of Cardiology* 41 (1978): 94.

32. Luderitz et al., "Therapeutic Pacing in Tachyarrythmias by Implanted Pacemakers."

33. M. Mirowski, M. Mower, W. Stawen, et al., "Standby Automatic Defibrillator." *Arch. Int. Med.* 126 (1970): 158; M. Mirowski, M. Mower, P. Reid, L.

Watkins, and A. Langer, "The Automatic Implantable Defibrillator." *PACE* 5, no. 3 (1982): 384; M. Mirowski, "An Automatic Implantable Pacemaker/Defibrillator." *Proc. 1st Andean Symposium on Pacemakers*, Bogata, Colombia, 1983.

34. Mirowski, "An Automatic Implantable Pacemaker/Defibrillator," 1983.

35. D. Duncan, B. Goldman, A. Chisholm, J. Pym, J. Cameron, E. Noble, A. Adelman, D. Cameron, and M. Waxman, "Initial Experience with Universal Pacemakers," *PACE* 6,no. 4 (1983): 806.

36. V. Parsonnet, S. Furman, and N. Smyth, "Implantable Cardiac Pacemakers: Status Report and Resource Guideline (ICHD)." *Circulation* 50 (1974): A21.

37. R. Hauser, "Resources Required for Pacemaker Implantation." *PACE* 6, no. 1 (1983): 139.

38. Parsonnet et al., "A Revised Code for Pacemaker Identification."

39. Furman, "Pacemaker Programmability."

40. P. Levine, P. Belott, M. Billitch, B. Boal, D. Escher, S. Furman, J. Griffin, R. Hauser, J. Maloney, D. Morse, and H. Semler, "Recommendations of the NASPE Policy Conference on Pacemaker Programmability and Follow-up." *PACE* 6, no. 6 (1983): 1222.

3

ELECTRODES AND LEADS

ELECTRODES IN BIOENGINEERING*

Much of the experimental work in this chapter was done in the author's personal laboratory in Clarence, New York, but much was also done in the chemistry department of Houghton College, in New York State. Many thanks are due to Bernard Piersma, Ph.D., Stephan Calhoun, Ph.D., and Frederick Shannon, Ph.D., for their help and for the use of their high-purity polarization facility.

Introduction

A physiological electrode is an electrochemical interface between living tissue and a machine. Its function is to transform biochemical and physiological phenomena into electrical currents, or, conversely, to generate such phenomena from electric currents.

Electricity flows through metallic conductors by electron flow, but flows through electrolytes such as body fluid or body tissue by ion flow. To transform electron current in a wire into ion flow in the body, a chemical reaction is necessary. This reaction takes place within a few angstroms of the metal surface and is usually a different reaction at the anode from that at the cathode.

---

*While the material is now twenty years old, much of it (especially the material on electrochemical polarization of physiological electrodes) is still contemporary. We must point out that newer electrode structures are not described here. Please refer to the appendix for this chapter at the back of this book for further information.

This article originally appeared in *CRC Critical Reviews in Bioengineering* 5, no. 1 (1981), CRC Press, Inc.

The reaction which takes place is a strong function of the metal used in the electrode. Depending on the metal used, the reaction responsible for current flow may well be a gas evolution, a gas adsorption or absorption, or a metal corrosion reaction. The science of physiological electrode reactions, even in pure media under laboratory conditions, is still a subject of much research and not completely understood. Obviously, to extend this science to physiological conditions introduces such a host of uncontrolled variables that one can usually only speak in generalities about the electrochemistry one will expect to see at the interface of a practical physiological electrode. Nevertheless, some very valuable conclusions can be drawn, and one can at least derive some strong conclusions about how some things should *not* be done.

In the first half of this century, active stimulation of tissue was largely confined to teaching and research situations, but in 1947 C. Beck et al. first demonstrated clinical cardiac defibrillation.[1] Then Paul Zoll in 1952 reported clinical use of an external cardiac stimulator.[2] In 1959 Wilson Greatbatch and William Chardack[3] reported the first implantable cardiac pacemaker, which was first successfully used clinically in the following year.[4] All of these devices used electricity in a pulsitile or AC form, as did numerous bladder stimulators for incontinence, carotid sinus nerve stimulators for alleviating hypertension, and implantable and transcutaneous nerve stimulators for alleviating intractable pain.

Direct current stimulation, with a whole new set of electrochemical problems, is coming into increased use in a new field. This is the electronic control of growth and of infection. I. Yasuda,[5] C. Brighton et al.,[6] and Becker and J. Spadero[7] have all demonstrated accelerated healing of broken bones by the use of DC electrical current in the 1 to 80 µA range. Spadero et al.[8] have demonstrated the killing of animal bacteria and the killing of certain floating tumors by positive currents of as little as 0.4 µA on silver electrodes. Greatbatch[9] has extended Spadero's work down to DC currents as low as 24 nA and applied this technique to the killing of plant bacteria and plant viroids. Work is underway to determine whether this same anodic silver lethality applies also to plant and animal viruses.

Thus, as always, the use of a new tool in the hands of avid experimenters has quickly transcended the understanding of why the tool works. It is indeed encouraging that so many established electrochemists —such as Brummer and Turner,[10] B. Piersma et al.,[11] A. Salkind,[12] and others—have directed much of their thinking towards the electrochemistry of the physiological electrode. It is only through such an approach that true understanding will evolve.

It might be well to mention briefly some of the desirable performance parameters. We seek such things as biocompatibility. We will say many times that the electrode must not poison the body and the body must not poison the electrode, either through electrochemical action or physiological rejection. Prompt tissue ingrowth in an implantable electrode is an important factor. Electrode instability, either mechanical or electrical, will lead to certain failure. Recent work has strongly emphasized this aspect of electrode design. We will also emphasize the dual nature of the bioelectrode as an electrochemical device and as a physiological device. One couples to the body, but the other either senses or elicits physiological function. One is purely electrochemical, but the other requires a living organism. Thus, polarization and stimulation threshold must not be confused.

In this chapter we approach metal electrodes from five aspects. First we discuss the origins of electrochemical potentials in the electrolyte environment. Following this we examine what happens when a metal is introduced into the electrolyte, both under static and under driven conditions. Next we consider structural aspects of clinical bioelectrodes; i.e., those used on or in patients. We consider both the lead, which merely carries the electrical signal to or from the electrode, and the electrode itself, which is that portion of the conducting system that electrically contacts the body.

Since most bioelectrodes are used on pacemakers, our treatment of the subject stresses this area. Other applications are considered, however, and a last section of this chapter is devoted to the emerging fields of osteogenesis and infection control.

This chapter is a coalescence of the author's fifty years of enjoyable experiences in this field, complete with some reminiscences, some biased opinions, and, hopefully, some useful information on some developments, new and old, that might not be readily available to some workers in the field.

The Electrolyte Environment

A. *Ions in Solution*

Ions in solution act both as conductors of electrical charge and to develop electric potentials at interfaces. Ions carry the charge in solution. They act as majority or minority carriers, depending on their relative concentration and the mobility of the individual species. In the body, sodium, chloride, and, in some cases, potassium ions are majority carriers. They are present in fairly large concentrations and are quite mobile. A minority carrier would be one with perhaps 5 percent or less of the concentration of a majority carrier. A minority ion carrier carries very little of the charge as current passes through tissue or electrolyte.

If one assumes that individual ions of a given species are so remote from each other that they do not affect each other, then the activity will be nearly equal to the concentration. Most body fluids are dilute enough to permit this assumption in biomedical work, but it is important to recognize that this may not be true in strong solutions (100 g/l of NaCl, for example).

Ions generate electric potentials at interfaces. The ion has two masters: concentration gradient and charge gradient. The ion as a chemical substance will move downhill from a concentration of like ions. Yet, as a charge carrier, the ion must respond to electric fields: like charges repelling like charges; opposite charges, attracting. The electric potentials generated by ions in solution result from the ion trying to respond to both masters at once.

B. *Membrane Potentials*

Consider two NaCl solutions of different concentrations, separated by a membrane permeable only to Na^+. The Na^+ ions on the stronger side will begin to migrate through the membrane to the weaker side. As they do, they will carry a positive charge to the weaker side, leaving a negative charge on the stronger. As this charge increases, it will begin to repel new Na^+ ions coming across until an equilibrium is reached where forces on the Na^+ ion due to the concentration gradient are just equal to the opposite forces on the charge gradient.

This potential is known as a "Nernst" relationship:[13]

$$E(volts) = -\frac{RT}{nF} \ln \frac{C1}{C2}$$

$$= -.059 \, \log \frac{C1}{C2} \quad (\text{at } 25°C \text{ for monovalent ions})$$

where R = the gas constant, T = absolute temperature, n = number of electrons transferred per ion, F = Faraday constant, and C_1/C_2 = concentrations of the species (assumed here to be nearly equal to the activities). (See Figure 1.)

C. *Liquid Junction Potentials*

Similar potentials can be developed at liquid junctions. Consider the orifice of a saline-filled glass pipette in a sink of water. Sodium and chloride ions have different mobilities resulting in unequal diffusion rates through the orifice. The sodium ion, although smaller, becomes hydrated, very sluggish, and immobile compared to the unencumbered chloride ions. Thus, a potential will develop between the outside of the pipette and its contents. This potential will rise until it is sufficiently high to repel additional chloride ions trying to cross the orifice, after which equilibrium will exist. It is interesting to note that such a liquid potential would not develop with potassium ions since they have about the same mobility as chloride ions (Figure 2).

A biological example of liquid junction potential is seen in ECG skin electrodes. The skin has an insulating layer consisting of keratin and epidermis. When electrode jelly is applied, liquid junction potentials develop. Modulations of this potential by pressure, motion, and so on produce ECG artifact. Puncturing the keratin and epidermis with a needle or by abrasion aborts the liquid junction potential, permitting artifact-free recording if one is also using a nonpolarizable skin electrode.

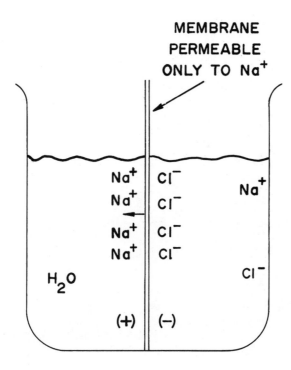

MEMBRANE PERMEABLE ONLY TO Na$^+$

Figure 1. Dynamic equilibrium of charge gradient versus concentration gradient across a membrane selectively permeable to Na$^+$ ions.

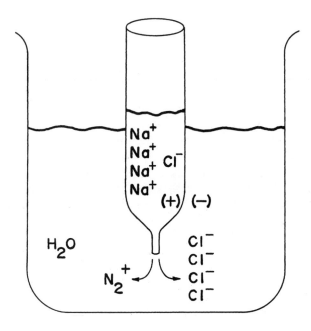

Figure 2. Dynamic equilibrium of charge gradient versus concentration gradient across a liquid junction due to ions of different mobility.

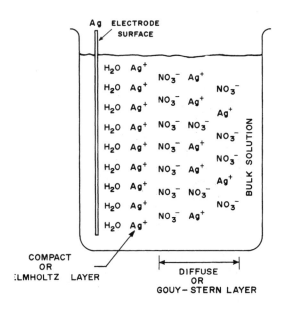

Figure 3. Formation of double-layer at a metal electrolyte interface.

Metal-Electrolyte Interface

A. Static Considerations

Let us consider a silver wire in a silver nitrate electrolyte solution. Electrons in the silver wire are majority carriers.

The silver and nitrate ions are majority carriers in the solution. They become arranged into an organized pattern in the vicinity of (within a few angstroms of) the electrode, and the silver wire begins reacting with the solution in a reversible reaction, i.e., $Ag \Leftrightarrow Ag^+ + e$. A dynamic equilibrium is reached at which point an excess of silver ions remains at the surface of the electrode forming the Helmholtz layer. An opposing layer with excess nitrate ions forms adjacent to the Helmholtz layer. This pattern is repeated with increasing disorder (the order diminishes exponentially with distance from the electrode surface) and forms the diffuse layer. The Helmholtz (or compact) layer and the diffuse layer are called the "electrical double layer" and exist at the surface of every metal-electrolyte interface. This charged layer is reversible and represents a significant part of the electrical capacitance of such an interface (see Figure 3).

The potential across this double-layer is the half-cell potential and is on the order of several hundred millivolts. At steady-state, the half-cell potential can be described by another form of the Nernst equation:

$$E_{Ag^+, Ag} = E^{\circ}_{Ag^+, Ag} + \frac{RT}{F} \ln A_{Ag^+}$$

$$E^{\circ}_{Ag^+, Ag} = 0.799 \text{ V}$$

plus a factor logarithmically related to the activity (concentration) of that ion.

If the solution does not contain an ion of the same metal, the Nernst voltage will be undefined and the electrode voltage will drift randomly. This will be true of a clean silver electrode immediately upon being placed in the body. If the electrode is coated with a layer of silver chloride, however, it will become a very stable bioelectrode with a resting potential within a millivolt of 222 mv above hydrogen. Such a coating is applied by electroplating or by mechanically compressing a mixture of pure silver and pure silver chloride powders into pellets. The intimate coating of silver chloride is a porous, nonconductive precipitate that is only sparingly soluble in water. This provides an environment of saturated solution at the metal surface. The concentration of silver ions at the electrode surface in this saturated solution is then dependent only on the concentration of chloride ions in the surrounding electrolyte, since:

$$K_{SP} = a_{Ag+}\, a_{Cl-}$$

where K_{SP} is the solubility product that is constant for a saturated solution at a given temperature. The chlorine ion concentration then determines the silver ion concentration. Thus, the silver chloride coating on the electrode interchanges charges with the sodium chloride environment via chloride and then interchanges charges with the silver electrode via silver. The resulting Nernst potential is then:

$$E_{AgCl,\, Ag,\, Cl-} = E^{\circ}{}_{A,Cl,Ag,Cl-} - \frac{RT}{F}\, \ln a_{Cl-}$$

The Nernst potential is now dependent only on absolute temperature and chloride activity. This says that for recording to be free of artifact, one must have a common ion across each chemical interface.

It is interesting to note that implanted silver wires will eventually become spontaneously chloridized, but imperfectly so. Thin chloride layers will spontaneously interchange some chloride ions with oxide ions and also sulphide ions in the electrolyte. The resulting coating will therefore be less than ideal and of marginal stability.[14] Motion of the electrolyte at the interface will temporarily disrupt the concentration of the species, resulting in motion artifact. It is common practice in ECG electrodes to protect the interface in a well or in a separate compartment or behind a fabric or sponge separator.

Many ECG electrodes today are one-time-use, throwaway types in which expensive manufacturing procedures are not possible. Such silver electrodes are usually merely plated or coated in some other manner. They far surpass the older bare metal electrodes but cannot compare to true silver-silver chloride pellet electrodes of the much more expensive Mennen Medical or Hewlett Packard types. The author has a set of 50 percent Ag/AgCl MG (now Mennen Medical) pellet electrodes that are now over 30 years old. When properly applied to the chest, they still give less than 1 mV artifact, even when sharply struck by the flat of the hand.

B. *Polarization*

The above considerations have applied to passive (undriven) electrodes. Additional potentials arise when electrodes are electrically driven. The term "polarization" sometimes means different things to different electrochemists, who often disagree on its definition. We will beg this issue here and merely describe it in terms of what happens in typical physiological electrode systems. For this it will suffice for us to consider only "ohmic" polarization and "concentration" polarization.

Ohmic polarization is that which behaves in accordance with Ohm's Law; i.e., it is resistive in nature. Oxide or chloride or organic coatings on the electrode surface can reduce effective surface area and modify the low resistance characteristics of the metal. Surface structures might enhance conductivity by increasing both porosity and effective surface area or might inhibit it by decreasing surface roughness. Any potential drop at the interface which is linearly and instantaneously related to current is then "ohmic." For physiological purposes, we will define "instantaneously" as that which happens in a few microseconds or less. Thus, ohmic polarization will reveal no apparent capacitive effects at frequencies of physiological interest. A square wave of current will elicit a square wave of voltage.

Concentration polarization, in contrast, presents a strong capacitive element. As current is driven through the electrode/electrolyte interface, and ions are either depleted or concentrated near the electrode surface. When the current is turned off, they diffuse back to an equilibrium state, but only after a period of some time. Thus, a potential is developed which is dependent on the time the current was on or off and on the magnitude of that current. This is particularly true of pacemaker electrodes.

Kenneth Cole[15] recognized the capacitive component at the interface nearly fifty years ago, but attributed it to the known high dielectric constant of the tissue cell membrane. It was not until the classic paper of P. Mansfield[16] and the subsequent work of J. Weinman and J. Mahler[17] and W. Greatbatch et al.[18] that it was recognized that the capacity has nothing whatsoever to do with the physiological life process and was truly only electrochemical in nature. Mansfield proved this by placing a micropipette against a metal plate. When perpendicular, the micropipette gave waveforms characteristic of the metal itself. When laid parallel to the plate, it gave waveforms characteristic of the solution. The transition from one situation to the other took place in a distance no greater than the diameter of the micropipette. This simple experiment completely changed the thinking of the early prosthetics experimenters with regard to electrode design.

The present author recollects the circumstances surrounding the publication of Mansfield's paper. It had been rejected by the journal's regular reviewers, but the editor, Paul Cranefield, referred it to me for a second opinion. I recommended it so strongly that the editor published it over the objections of the original referees.

In each person's life there are certain actions that one feels very good about. This is one of mine.

1. Properties of Platinum Electrodes

Newly implanted electrodes require a few weeks to stabilize, for tissue ingrowth, etc. We consider a mature electrode to be one that is six months old, or more.

Figure 4 shows the voltage waveform developed by a constant current pulse on a mature clinical myocardial electrode pair, both in a patient and in a saline bath. It is apparent that the capacitive properties are nearly identical.

Figure 5 shows the voltage developed across the interface of platinum pacemaker electrodes in 37°C physiological saline when driven by constant-current (galvanostatic) pulses of pacemaker duration (1.6 msec). DC steady-state baseline has been deleted. Several facts are immediately obvious. First, the load is capacitive in nature. A square-wave of current elicits an exponentially rising voltage. The rise-times of leading and trailing edge are very fast — a few microseconds at most.

Electrical charge is equal to the product of current and time and also to the product of capacity and voltage. Thus:

$$EC = Q = It$$

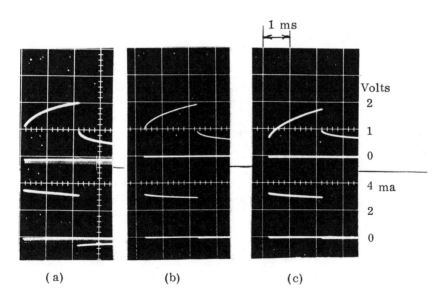

Figure 4. Voltage waveforms developed by a constant-current pulse on (a) a patient, (b) identical electrode in a 37°C saline bath, and (c) a similar electrode, unwound into a 2cm x 0.010"D cylinder, in a saline bath.

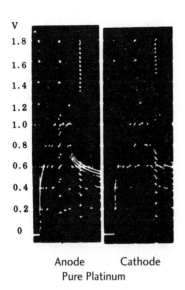

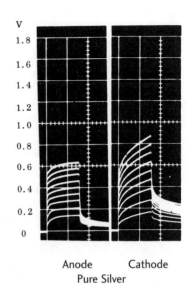

Anode   Cathode
Pure Platinum

Anode   Cathode
Pure Silver

Figure 5. Galvanostatic voltage waveforms on platinum anode and cathode developed by constant-current pulses of 1 to 9 mA.

Figure 6. Galvanostatic voltage waveforms on silver anode and cathode developed by constant-current pulses of 1 to 9 mA.

At the lowest level of 1mA for 1.6 msec (1.6 µC), the 0.2 V rise implies an effective capacity of 8 µF, a sizable capacity indeed.

One notes also that a postpulse charge remains on the electrode surface long after the pulse has ceased. As one increases the pulse amplitude in steps from 1 to 9 mA, the postpulse charge increases also, although somewhat less than linearly. We note, too, the nearly identical waveform pattern for anode and cathode. No other metal has this latter characteristic.

2. Properties of Silver Electrodes

In contrast, in Figure 6 the silver electrode anode presents a very low voltage drop with negligible postpulse charge. The silver anode becomes chloridized by the positive pulses and thus behaves much like a silver-silver chloride reference electrode. On the cathode any residual chloride actually becomes stripped off, leaving bare metal which is highly polarizable. Thus the cathode does reveal an exponentially rising voltage and a postpulse charge.

It is interesting to note that the stripping off of the spontaneous chloridization can be easily seen. Figure 7 shows the stripping taking place over a period of 2 ½ hours of pulsing at 3.3 mA per 2.6 msec pulse, once each second.

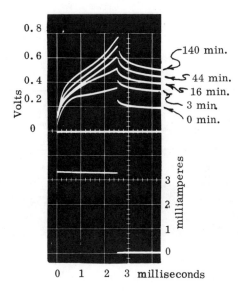

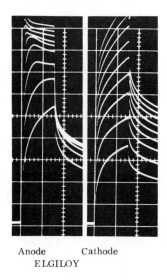

Figure 7. Increasing polarization on a silver cathode versus time showing stripping off of the nonpolarizable chloride layer.

Figure 8. Galvanostatic voltage waveforms on Elgiloy anode and cathode developed by constant-current pulses of 1 to 9 mA.

3. Behavior of Stainless Steel and Cobalt Alloys

Next let us consider the behavior of Elgiloy (a common cardiac electrode metal), under these same conditions. In Figure 8 we note first that the same current levels that were used in Figure 5 elicit far higher voltages. That is to say, it is necessary to have a far greater driving voltage to get the same current to flow. This is, of course, an energy loss indicating that such an electrode system is far less efficient than platinum or silver. One notes, too, the aberrant waveform on the anode. There are clearly some complex reactions going on during the 1.6 msec duration of the pulse. The postpulse charge has an interesting pattern. Note that the postpulse pattern is clearly apparent for 1, 2, 3, and 4 mA pulses, but at 5, 6, 7, 8, and 9 mA they are all superimposed and indistinguishable. We suspect that this unexpected energy loss is going into some degree of electrode corrosion. Under these same stimulation conditions, we have used spectraphotometric analysis to detect chromium and cobalt ions in solution after stimulating stainless steel, Elgiloy, and MP 35 anodes. In similar tests, we have looked for and found corrosion by-products from platinum and titanium electrodes, but to find the latter it has been necessary to resort to atomic absorption techniques. Platinum and titanium residues have been 1,000 times less than found with any of the nonnoble metals.

It may well be that the levels of corrosion we see are not significant in the normal pacemaker system lifetime, but one should recognize that they do exist and are measurable.

Complementing the above work, we have published our waveform patterns and our chemical analysis on a dozen or more commonly used electrode metals and alloys.[19] (See Figures 9, 10, and 11.)

C. *Coupling Reactions*

It was previously mentioned that majority electron flow in metals can become ion flow in electrolytes only through a chemical reaction at the metal surface. The reaction that takes place will depend on the ionic species present in the electrolyte, the metal in the electrode, and the voltage available. If the electrode metal does not have the same ion present in the electrolyte, the potential will drift randomly until driven to a point where some other species in the electrolyte will react. Hydrogen will be generated at a level of 0.000v on the Reversible Hydrogen Scale. Silver chloride can form at + 0.222v above hydrogen. Monatomic oxygen can form and adsorb catalytically on platinum at + 0.9v versus hydrogen and can evolve as a diatomic gas at + 2v or so. S. Brummer and M. Turner[20] and others teach that oxygen adsorbed on platinum forms as platinum oxide rather than monatomic oxygen as believed by Bernard

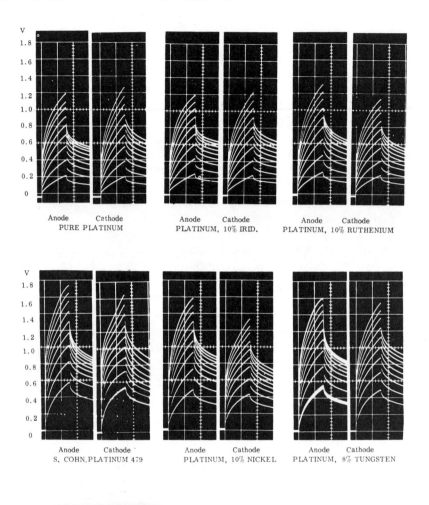

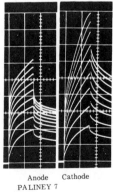

Figure 9. Galvanostatic voltage waveforms on a number of platinum alloys, developed by constant-current pulses of 1 to 9 mA. (From W. Greatbatch et al., *Ann. N.Y. Acad. Sci.* 167, no. 2, 722, 1969.)

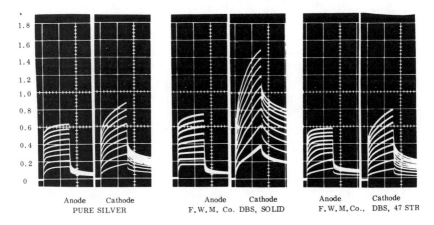

Figure 10. Galvanostatic voltage waveforms on a number of silver structures and alloys, developed by constant-current pulses of 1 to 9 mA. (From W. Greatbatch et al., *Ann. N.Y. Acad. Sci.* 167, no. 2, 722, 1969.)

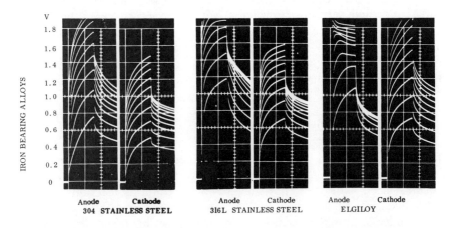

Figure 11. Galvanostatic voltage waveforms on a number of iron-cobalt-chromium alloys, developed by constant-current pulses of 1 to 9 mA. (From W. Greatbatch et al., *Ann. N.Y. Acad. Sci.* 167, no. 2, 722, 1969.)

Piersma et al.[21] and T. Warner et al.[22] The difference is probably academic, and the author knows no way of experimentally resolving the issue. At more positive voltages, chlorine can evolve, and metallic corrosion of stainless steel can take place.

The threshold voltages of such reactions are not precise values. The actual electrode voltage will depend on at least three factors.

First, the magnitude of driven current will have some effect on the overvoltage needed to drive the reaction. A very small current will require very little overvoltage; a larger current will require more overvoltage.

Second, some reaction will actually proceed at zero net current flow. Zero net current does not mean zero local currents. There will always be some exchange current backward and forward between metal and electrolyte; for example, between silver and silver chloride and between silver chloride and chloride ion in a saline electrolyte. In the latter example, these exchange currents will come to equilibrium at an electrode voltage of 222 mv above hydrogen. If a very small current is now driven through the electrode, it will not appear as a new current where there was zero current before, but rather as a modification of the equilibrium of exchange current. This small current may not be able to strip a silver wire clean of chloride. Rather, some small amount of chloride may continue to be formed by the exchange current, holding the electrode at the silver chloride potential, even in the face of a small negative current.

Third, in a real-life, dirty electrolyte system such as the human body, organics or other contaminants can easily poison electrode surfaces, modifying their behavior from what would be seen in pure laboratory electrolyte systems. Such poisoning need not incapacitate the electrode systems, but may well cause them to behave in unpredictable ways. The real-life operation of pacemaking electrode systems and other such prosthetic electrodes must accommodate such variables. They are probably best studied in the real-life situation.

1. Platinum Metal-Electrolyte Reactions

Bernard Piersma et al. have intensively studied the behavior of the platinum surface when pulsed in high-purity physiological saline under pacemaker conditions.[23] They find the major coupling reaction to be a reversible catalytic adsorption of monatomic oxygen on the metal surface. Added to this are minor contributions from hydrogen desorption, double-layer charging, and chlorine evolution, depending on the magnitude and duration of the pulse. Platinum is catalytic to oxygen and will spontaneously pick up a stored charge at higher potentials of up to 1300 $\mu C/cm^2$. In magnitude, such a charge is enough of a reservoir to supply several pacemaker impulses without replenishing. Thus it represents a capacitor storage of considerable magnitude, much more than that available from any other pacemaker electrode metal.

The resting potential of platinum at 37°C open to the atmosphere appears to be 0.80 to 0.85v above hydrogen, due to the spontaneous catalytic adsorption of monatomic O atoms.

Figure 12 shows a typical high-current (400 mA/cm²) anodic charging curve for platinum in a high-purity system, sealed away from ambient air.[24]

2. Silver Metal-Electrolyte Reactions

A silver wire in saline electrolyte will become coated with silver chloride to some degree. When such an electrode is driven negative, it will drive down to the hydrogen potential of 0 volts (by definition). At that point, some hydrogen will begin to evolve. It may not be visible as gas bubbles. If the current is very small, in the microampere range, or of very short duration, the gas may be adsorbed or dissolved in the electrolyte as fast as it is generated. If the voltage is driven very far below zero volts, much more hydrogen will be evolved, even though the overvoltage may be only a few tenths of a volt below zero. There will be no appreciable corrosion of the metal since it will be "cathodically protected."

If the silver wire is driven positive, another barrier will be reached at + 0.222v where silver chloride will form. This is a corrosion reaction which will eventually destroy the structural integrity of the metal electrode.

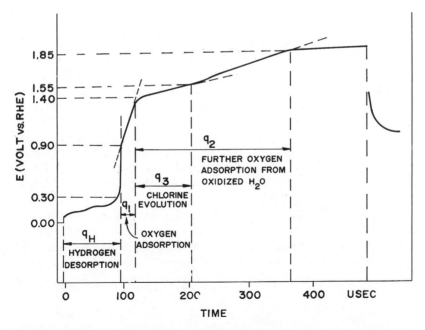

Figure 12. Typical high-current charging curve on platinum in an ultrapure saline system. Note the four sequential chemical reactions taking place in less than half a millisecond.

Thus the normal range of voltage over which the silver electrode can be driven is between zero volts and + 0.222v, plus whatever overvoltage is necessary to support the driving current. In bone growth and infection control stimulators, operating at 10 μA DC or less, we have rarely seen overvoltages of more than 0.2v above and below the 0 to + 0.222v range.

Recently, we have begun to use a new electrode metal which is 90 percent silver and 10 percent palladium. This alloy approaches the strength of pure platinum and is several times stronger than pure silver. An added advantage is the fact that palladium is catalytic to hydrogen so that less overvoltage is required when driving negatively to get the same desired current.

By limiting the palladium content to 10 percent, corrosion of the wire is not appreciably inhibited. Such corrosion is necessary when silver anodes are used as silver ion sources for infection control.[25] Increasing the palladium content to 25 percent tends to inhibit anodic corrosion, if this is desirable, and will add some strength. Table 4 (later in the chapter) shows comparative strengths of the above metals.

3. Titanium Metal-Electrode Reactions

Titanium, although rarely used now as a myocardial or endocardial pacemaker electrode, is commonly used as a large-area indifferent electrode, as a pacemaker enclosure. In past years, this metal was used as a pacemaker electrode with good results. We believe it to be electrochemically attractive in this service. Titanium cathodes seem to couple through the very high dielectric constant of the oxide coating on the metal surface. The electrode behaves as a highly efficient leaky capacitor, which may have a voltage drop a little larger than that of platinum.

On the anode side, titanium is less efficient and seems to operate on gas evolution of oxygen. However, since the anode is generally a large-area pacemaker enclosure, the current density will be a fraction of that at the cathode, and the polarization voltage loss will again be low. We find titanium corrosion reactions to be several times that of platinum, but a thousand times less than that of stainless steel or the iron-cobalt alloys.

C. Hall and J. Hackerman state that the original anodic polarization of titanium requires 360 times as much charge as a subsequent repolarization. They suggest an irreversible chemisorption of an 85 percent monolayer of oxygen atoms.[26]

Piersma et al. find the subsequent transfer reaction to be wholly accountable to charging of the double layer by O_2 evolution on the anode and H_2 evolution on the cathode.[27] The resting potential of titanium electrodes is always within 25 mv of hydrogen, indicating that titanium adsorbs helium much as palladium does. Even after purging with helium, titanium retains its hydrogen potential (and its hydrogen atoms) much longer than platinum.

4. Stainless Steel and Iron-Cobalt Metal Electrode Reactions

The stainless steel and cobalt alloys all operate on surface reactions which are much less efficient than the platinum and silver metals. There is always some corrosion measurable on the anode electrode, although it may be small enough to be negligible over the life of the system. Such metals are used because of their strength. Platinum and silver metals, while electrochemically more attractive, are not strong enough to support a temporary stiffening stylet in a helical lead. For this reason, the stainless steel and cobalt alloys are nearly universally used for the leads of permanent transvenous endocardial pacemaker catheters.

These alloys are not catalytic to any gas reactions, and they do not form efficient chloride coatings, as does silver. Rather they operate between hydrogen evolution at zero volts and oxygen evolution at about + 2v. There is a minor cushion of double-layer charge capacity which can assist in the coupling mechanism, but it is only a fraction of that present on the platinum electrode. On the positive side, some metal corrosion will always be found. To minimize such corrosion, nonnoble anodes should never be used as small-area myocardial or endocardial pairs against a similar cathode structure. The anode should rather be a large-area indifferent electrode, such as the metal pacemaker enclosure. By so reducing the current density at the metal surface, corrosion reactions can be minimized.

D. *Energy Losses in Cardiac Electrodes as a Function of Pulse Length*

Geoffrey Davies and Edgar Sowton[28] have shown that the threshold of cardiac stimulation is directly related to the product of the voltage, the current, and the time duration of the impulse applied through metal electrodes to the heart. Thus, threshold stimulation is a linear function of the energy content of the pulse over a wide range of pulse lengths.

Our own group confirmed Davies's work on platinum electrodes and found that this relationship extends from pulse durations below 0.3 msec to over 4.0 msec,[29] particularly if electrode polarization losses are taken into account. Our method of isolating polarization losses was to calculate total energy consumption as the product of average values of time, voltage, and current but to calculate the energy delivered to the load using leading-edge values of voltage and current. We used a pulse generator that was nearly constant-current. We hypothesized that the leading-edge values represented energy actually delivered to the load all during the pulse, while the rising voltage during the pulse represented power loss due to polarizing the electrode. We assumed that ohmic polarization of the interface could be neglected.

Table 1 shows the raw data from which Figures 13 to 16 are drawn. Table 2 shows some additional data taken on a pair of mature platinum myocardial electrodes on a canine heart. Even without allowance for electrode polarization losses, the relative independence of energy threshold on pulse duration is obvious. Table 3 shows threshold data on 11 patients taken at the time of pacemaker pulse generator replacement. Data were taken at two pulse lengths, 0.8 and 2.0 msec. It will be noticed that there is no significant difference between energy thresholds at the two pulse durations.

Figure 13 shows the familiar strength-duration plot of threshold current versus pulse duration. Figure 14 shows the same data with average voltage included and plotted as energy versus pulse duration. One will note that replotting in terms of energy flattens the curve out quite considerably. Figure 15 represents the electrode polarization energy losses which when subtracted from the total energy in Figure 14 gives the actual physiological energy-duration curve with electrode effects removed.

When considering such curves, it is essential to keep in mind which components of this problem are electrochemical and which are physiological. Stimulation threshold is a physiological parameter. It is the least value of energy (or charge or current or voltage) to which the heart will physiologically respond. Polarization is an electrochemical parameter and defines how much voltage drop will exist for a given current condition. The two are not the same. One can get polarization data from a saline bath, but threshold stimulation can only be determined on a physiological preparation of some kind. (See Figure 16.)

These three sets of data give strong support to Geoffrey Davies's findings that the one parameter which determines stimulation threshold is energy rather than charge, current, or voltage.

E. *Faradaic Rectification*

In order to identify the reactions which take place at the electrode interface, it is necessary to know the region of the charging curve through which the electrode operates. The starting point may well be near the resting potential of the electrode at the first impulse, but each successive impulse will start from a different point. The reason for this is the fact that the reactions at the positive excursion of the electrode are different from those at the negative excursion. Thus, a rectification takes place which charges the capacity of the interface and displaces the next starting

TABLE 1
THRESHOLD ENERGY VERSUS PULSE DURATION ON A MATURE BIPOLAR TRANSVENOUS PLATINUM ELECTRODE PAIR

Pulse duration (msec)	LEA/TEA[a] (volts)	Average	LEA/TEA[a] (mA)	Average	Total[b]	Load[c]	Polarization loss (μj)
4.00	0.50/0.90	0.70	1.4/ 1.3	1.35	3.8	2.8	1.0
3.00	0.55/0.90	0.73	1.6/ 1.5	1.55	3.4	2.6	0.8
2.00	0.65/1.0	0.83	2.1/ 2.0	2.05	3.4	2.7	0.7
1.50	0.75/1.1	0.93	2.3/ 2.1	2.20	3.1	2.6	0.5
1.00	0.8 /1.2	1.00	2.5/ 2.4	2.45	2.5	2.0	0.5
0.75	1.0 /1.4	1.20	3.0/ 3.0	3.00	2.8	2.3	0.5
0.50	1.3 /1.6	1.45	3.7/ 3.7	3.70	2.7	2.4	0.3
0.30	1.8 /2.1	1.95	5.0/ 5.0	5.00	2.9	2.7	0.2
0.20	2.5 /2.9	2.70	7.5/ 7.5	7.50	4.1	3.8	0.3
0.10	3.5 /4.4	3.95	12 /12	12.00	4.7	4.2	0.5

Note: (Dog 57, p3b 277 Aug. 19, 1966). Electrode area tip, 0.855 cm^2; ring, 0.805 cm^2; implanted 6 months, Medtronic 5816.
[a] LEA/TEA, leading edge amplitude/trailing edge amplitude.
[b] Total energy, $V_{avg} \times I_{avg} \times t$.
[c] Load energy, $V_{LEA} \times I_{LEA} \times t$.

TABLE 2
THRESHOLD ENERGY VERSUS PULSE DURATION ON A MATURE MYOCARDIAL PAIR OF PLATINUM 10% IRIDIUM ELECTRODES IMPLANTED 6 MONTHS

Pulse duration (msec)	TEA[a] (volts)	TEA[a] (ma)	Energy (μJ)
0.1	5.1	10	5.1
0.2	3.0	5.2	3.1
0.3	2.5	4.0	3.0
0.4	2.0	3.0	2.4
0.5	2.4	1.7	2.0
0.7	1.5	2.0	2.1
1.0	1.5	1.9	2.85
1.5	1.2	1.3	2.35
2.0	1.05	0.9	1.90

Note: (Dog 715, p3B234, November 30, 1965). Trailing edge amplitudes only. Electrode area, 0.16 cm^2 ea. Medtronic 5814.
[a] TEA, trailing edge amplitude.

TABLE 3

DATA ON 11 PATIENTS WITH MATURE PLATINUM BIPOLAR ENDOCARDIAL MEDTRONIC 5816
ELECTRODES AT CONSTANT-CURRENT PULSES OF 2.0 AND 0.8 MSEC DURATION

| | Data at 2.0 msec | | | | Data at 0.8 msec | | | |
| | LEA/TEA[a] | | | Pulse energy | LEA/TEA[a] | | | Pulse energy |
Patient Number	(mA)	(volts)	Average	(μJ)	(mA)	(volts)	Average	(μJ)
1	3.7	1.0 /1.8	1.4	10.40	6.2	2.0/2.50	2.25	11.11
2	3.4	0.5 /1.0	0.75	5.10	5.8	1.0/1.25	1.13	5.25
3	3.6	0.6 /1.0	0.80	5.75	5.9	1.0/1.4	1.20	5.65
4	2.1	1.0 /1.4	1.20	5.05	3.8	1.7/2.0	1.85	5.63
5	2.5	1.0 /1.5	1.25	6.25	3.9	1.5/2.0	1.75	5.45
6	2.2	0.5 /0.8	0.65	2.86	3.6	0.8/1.3	1.05	3.02
7	6.0	1.8 /2.2	2.00	24.00	9.0	2.5/3.0	2.75	19.60
8	2.1	0.8 /1.0	0.90	3.78	4.4	1.2/1.8	1.50	5.28
9	5.6	1.0 /1.2	1.50	12.30	8.5	2.0/2.5	2.25	15.25
10	3.1	1.0 /2.0	1.50	9.30	5.1	2.0/2.5	2.25	9.18
11	4.3	1.5 /2.0	1.75	15.10	8.0	2.5/3.0	2.75	17.50
Mean	3.4	0.97/1.57	1.25	9.49	5.7	1.7/2.1	1.90	9.36

Note: Electrode area tip, 0.855 cm^2; ring, 0.805 cm^2.
[a]LEA/TEA, leading edge amplitude/trailing edge amplitude.

point of each excursion. If the rectification is stronger on the positive excursion, the subsequent starting potential will be driven negative. If the rectification is stronger on the negative excursion, the starting potential will be driven positive. Platinum has a resting potential in 37°C saline of 0.80 to 0.85v above hydrogen, but a repetitively negatively driven platinum cathode will start from above this point and drive down through monatomic oxygen desorption, through double-layer charging, and perhaps through hydrogen adsorption. We believe the principal means of coupling to be monatomic adsorption/desorption of oxygen. Once again, the presence of organics and other contaminants in the human physiological system may considerably distort this picture.

Kenneth Cole was the first to suggest that unwanted reactions such as metal corrosion and tissue necrosis could be minimized by ensuring that the net current flowing into an electrode is zero.[30] All modern pacemaking systems accomplish this by placing a high-quality capacitor electrically in series with the electrode lead. Such a capacitor is desirable, but does not unequivocally ensure that corrosion will not take place. Even though a capacitor is used, Faradaic rectification will ensure that part of the electrode excursion is into the corrosion region of nonnoble metals.

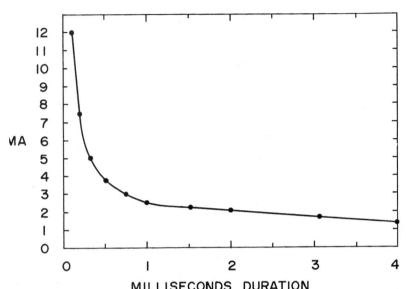

Figure 13. Conventional current versus duration curve on mature platinum endocardial catheter, plotted from data in Table 1.

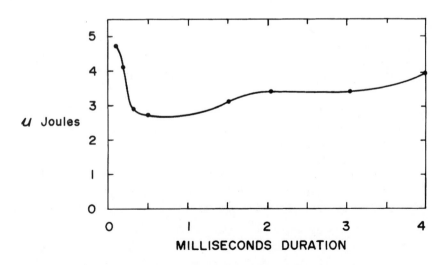

Figure 14. Energy versus duration curve on the electrode in Figure 13, plotted from data in Table 1.

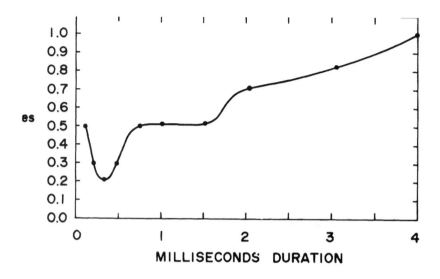

Figure 15. Energy loss at electrode surface of electrode in Figure 14, plotted from data in Table 1. Note the greatly expanded energy scale.

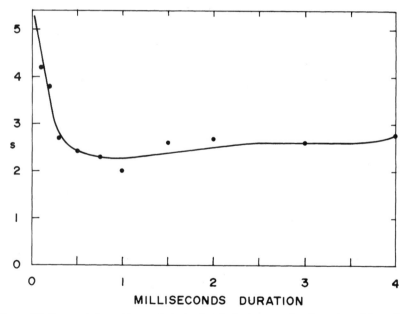

Figure 16. Energy delivered beyond electrode interface versus duration, plotted from data in Table 1. Allowing for electrode surface losses makes the energy versus duration curve very flat from 0.3 to 4 msec.

Early pacemaker experience with corrosion of the Hunter-Roth (Figure 21) anode[31] and of other such small-area nonnoble myocardial pairs demonstrated the fallacy of such an assumption. If a nonnoble metal is used as an anode, it must be a large-area plate to hold the corrosion current-density at the interface to a minimum.

STRUCTURAL ASPECTS OF THE CLINICAL BIOELECTRODE

A. *Historical Notes*

One of the early clinical uses of bioelectrodes was in the treatment of acute heart block in infants and children. With the advent of open heart surgery in the 1950s, the repair of septal defects in children became common. Some such defects were found lying close to the atrio-ventricular bundle of nerves, which traverses the septum carrying the "beat" signal from the atrium to the ventricle. Surgical repair sometimes inadvertently resulted in surgical disruption of the bundle, resulting in heart block. Such block, while often fatal in outcome, was nevertheless an acute situation, and Lillehei et al.[32] in Minneapolis conceived the idea of leaving one or more stainless steel wires sewn to the myocardium and brought outside the body. This permitted attachment of a small, wearable transistorized pacemaker, designed by Earl Bakken,[33] to support the child during periods of arrest.

Such wires were temporary in nature and were only meant to overcome the surgical trauma during the first few postoperative weeks. It was soon found, however, that if normal heart function did not return within three weeks, permanent stimulation would be necessary. Even though the child might regain normal heart function in two months, the result would be 100 percent fatal within one year without long-term stimulation. Weirich's[34] electrodes were not strong enough to withstand long-term fatigue. Samuel Hunter et al.[35] then designed a braided stainless steel lead terminating in a stainless steel myocardial pin encased in a silicone rubber patch. Such electrodes were used in pairs, sutured to the epicardium with the steel spike penetrating the myocardium.

Hunter's electrodes were extensively used by C. Walton Lillehei for longer term stimulation of patients in permanent, complete block. They were also the electrodes used by the present author's team in the first implantable pacemaker[36] and also in the first few clinical pacemakers implanted by our group[37] (see Figure 17).

The weak point of these early electrodes, which eventually led to the cessation of their use, was the corrosion of the small-area stainless steel

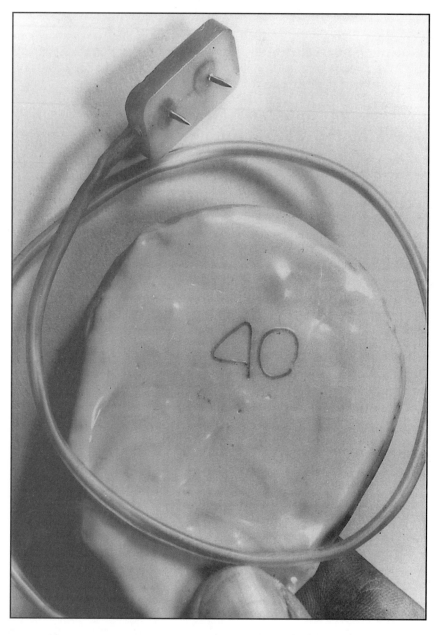

Figure 17. Hunter Roth myocardial electrode with early 10-cell, Chardack-Greatbatch (Medtronic 5850) pulse generator. The output of this pacemaker was a 13.5 V (open circuit), 2 msec pulse.

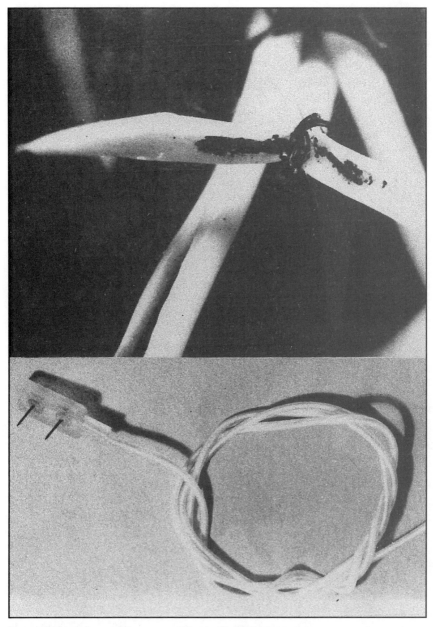

Figure 18. Anodic corrosion on an early Hunter Roth electrode.

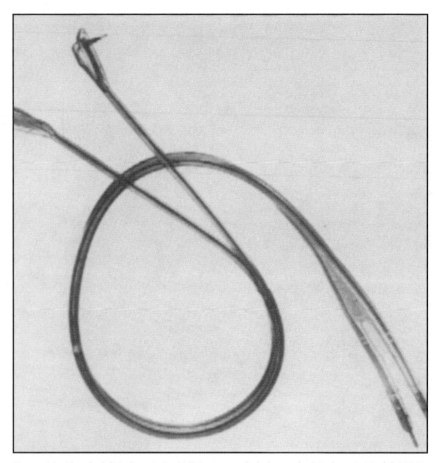

Figure 19. Chardack/Medtronic Pt 10% Ir myocardial electrode (Medtronic Model 5814). This was the first spring-coil platinum electrode.

anode (Figure 18). The anode lead and/or the anode pin would corrode away in a matter of months, causing a cessation of pacemaker function.

Chardack[38] then developed a new electrode concept which attacked both the electrical corrosion aspect and the mechanical fatigue aspect of the problem. His solution was a noble metal electrode and lead which was wound in the form of a spring coil. The lead terminated in an extended portion of the spring held in a perforated silicone rubber patch. The metal was an alloy of platinum-iridium with a yield strength of well over 100,000 psi (see Figure 19 and Figure 20).

In the meantime, Dr. Hans Lagergren[39] and associates in Stockholm had developed a very finely braided stainless steel wire which terminated

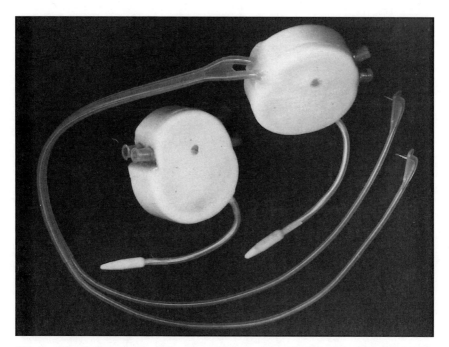

Figure 20. Early Chardack-Greatbatch/Medtronic 5860 pulse generator with Chardack/Medtronic Model 5814 myocardial electrode.

in a very small stainless steel tip. Since it was European practice to use unipolar systems (a stimulating cathode against a large-area indifferent anode), Hunter's corrosion problems did not come into play.

All early pacemaker systems used a thoracotomy approach with myocardial or epicardial electrodes, sewn directly on the surface of the heart. The trauma of the thoracotomy, along with the necessary general anesthesia, resulted in a rather universal 10 percent early mortality on these older, poor-risk patients. Seymour Furman and J. Schwedel[40] had early used external transvenous catheters for temporary heart pacing, thus avoiding the thoracotomy and the general anesthesia. Chardack[41] designed a spring-coil bipolar catheter with a temporary stylet for permanent implantable use. This catheter, which eventually was copied by many others, was—to a large degree—the approach of choice for over a decade (see Figure 21).

More recently there has been a tendency to return to the older myocardial techniques with a "limited thoracotomy" approach. The heart is exposed through a very small approach. A special "screw-in" electrode is passed down to the epicardium on the end of a nylon holder. It is then literally screwed into the myocardium, after which the nylon

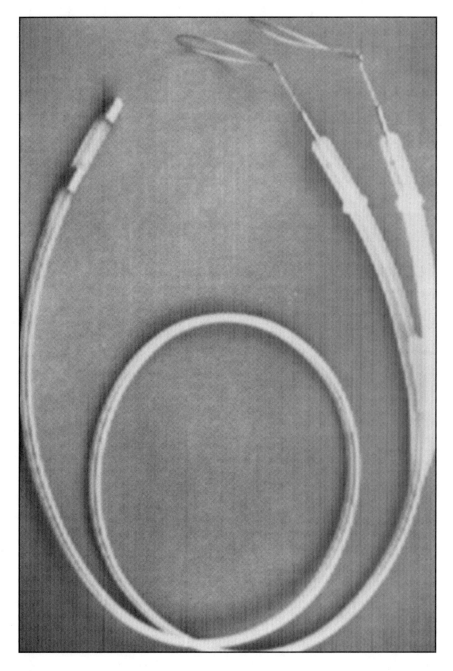

Figure 21. Early Chardack/ Medtronic Pt transvenous endocardial catheter electrode (Medtronic Model 5816).

holder is separated from the electrode and backed off. Such an approach obtains the advantages of direct myocardial stimulation, but avoids the potential problems of having heart valves continually closing around the endocardial catheter lead. Problems from this source have been gratifyingly rare, but some have been reported. (See Figure 22.)

B. *General Structural Considerations*

The physiological electrode operates in an intensely hostile environment, far more stringent in many ways than outer space or the bottom of the sea. The electrode must survive constant flexing (some 30 million c/year in a cardiac electrode) in a warm, corrosive, saline media. The materials used must be inert, not subject to fatigue, and must not produce unwanted physiological effects or chemical effects on the host media.

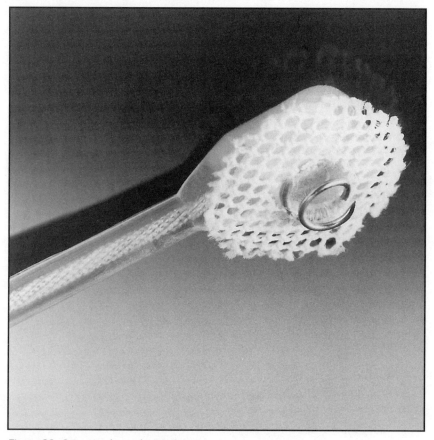

Figure 22. Screw-in electrode (Medtronic).

The most inert materials are platinum conductors and silicone rubber insulators. Unfortunately, pure platinum is not particularly strong, but when alloyed with iridium, it becomes stronger than structural steel. Silver is a very attractive metal in certain circumstances, but pure silver is even softer than platinum. However, when silver is alloyed with 10 percent palladium, it becomes three times as strong as it is in the pure state.

Table 4 presents a comparison of the relative strength of the above silver and platinum alloys as tested on an Instron tensile strength test machine.

Platinum can be alloyed with up to 40 percent of iridium without noticeably affecting its electrochemical properties. When alloyed with 25 percent palladium, silver becomes much less corrosive and loses its usefulness as a silver ion generator for infection control.

Alloying with up to 10 percent palladium, however, triples the strength of pure silver, but still permits it to ionize in saline when anodically driven, thus keeping its germicidal value.

C. Unipolar versus Bipolar Considerations

A bipolar structure has more or less identical anode and cathode structures. Either can stimulate although the physiological threshold will be 15 percent lower at the cathode. A unipolar structure consists of a single stimulating electrode (invariably a cathode) and a large-area indifferent anode, which is usually the metallic pacemaker enclosure. Both systems have seen extensive use, the unipolar being seen more in Europe and the bipolar being more common in the United States.

Historically, the early work of Dr. William Chardack[42] suggested that bipolar structures approached a stable value of threshold stimulation in about

TABLE 4
RELATIVE STRENGTHS OF 0.010"D PURE SILVER,
PURE PLATINUM, AND TWO OF THEIR ALLOYS

Material	Yield strength (0.2% elongation) (psi)	Tensile strength (rupture point) (psi)	Elongation at rupture (%)
Pure silver	14,013	23,822	26.6
Pure platinum	61,431	65,805	1.3
Silver 10% palladium	91,274	116,300	5.1
Platinum 10% iridium	113,916	118,290	1.5
Lot 2936			
Lot 4497	113,121	157,853	7.3

three weeks, whereas unipolar electrodes continued to increase in threshold indefinitely. It was subsequently found that their unipolar data were complicated by infection, but by then the pattern had been set and most subsequent American work was bipolar. European experience with unipolar electrodes was good. The reliability of the Siemans Elema/Lagergren electrode proved excellent, and most European work continues to be unipolar.

Actually, there are advantages to both systems. The fact that after twenty years of pacemaking neither system has become exclusively used proves that each system has good properties which still attract adherents.

The unipolar system is a much smaller, more innocuous structure. It is probably somewhat less traumatic to the heart valves that close around it, although this does not appear to be a problem area. For those who like to use waveform analysis of a pacemaker pulse, the unipolar system will give much more readable signals. The bipolar system is almost self-shielding in this regard. Both systems probably have equally low stimulation thresholds. Some say that the short separation of anode and cathode makes the bipolar pair less effective, but in fact one can often see greater amplitudes of endocardial QRS due to the fact that a QRS wave progressing across the heart can drive one electrode negative and the other positive, essentially doubling the amplitude of the sensed signal. One might think that a single polarity QRS wave in the same plane as the electrodes could give a zero signal, since the electrodes see only differences. However, to achieve cancellation, both the amplitude and the phase of the two electrode signals would have to be precisely equal. The probability of this happening is very low. The author can remember only two instances in twenty years of work where this has actually happened, one in an animal and one in a patient.

The bipolar system is inherently redundant. Should one lead break, the system is rather easily converted to unipolar by using the remaining good wire as a unipolar cathode and adding a large-area indifferent anode plate at some subcutaneous site. The bipolar system is an order of magnitude less susceptible to outside interference from external electrical signals or from local muscle potentials.

D. *The Lead*

A pacemaker system consists of a pulse generator, a lead wire, and an electrode. In accordance with electrochemical usage, an electrode is that portion of the metallic system in contact with the electrolyte. The purpose of the lead is to conduct the electrical impulse to the electrode. It must be strong, flexible, noncorrosive, and a good electrical conductor. Most design innovations have attacked one or more of these four aspects of lead design. One fundamental principle of lead design is that the wire must never be stretched beyond its elastic limit. Any repetitive fatigue flexing that even slightly exceeds the elastic limit will result in a "necking down" of the strained section. The section will then inevitably fail, sooner or later, depending only on the degree of the repeated strain. Soft flaccid metals therefore have no place in leads or electrodes. The metals must be as hard and as flexible as can possibly be obtained. Any stretching at all, if repetitive, will result in breakage. Some feel that it is satisfactory to place a highly conductive but soft material like pure silver in a stiff sheath and allow the silver to bend plastically inside the stiff sheath, which then supplies the strength. This is an erroneous concept since the plastic bending of the silver will destroy it even though the stiff sheath survives.

1. Braided Leads

Early work utilized leads of many strands, twisted or braided. Some contemporary designs still use this approach. We have already mentioned the Siemans Elema structure, which is simple and reliable. The placing of such an electrode requires the use of a stylet which surrounds the catheter. This requires a technique that is not easily acquired. Most American doctors do not favor it, but it is a very popular technique in Europe, where it is commonly and successfully used. Such electrodes are supplied without a terminating connector at the end proximal to the pulse generator. The lead is cut to the desired length and then inserted into the pulse generator where the polyethylene insulating sheath is punctured by a pointed stainless steel set screw which contacts the central braided cable and makes electrical contact. Some "screw-in" electrode designs also utilize a braided lead, but with a conventional connector.

2. Spring Coil Myocardial Leads

The first successful permanent pacemaker lead was the Chardack/ Medtronic myocardial electrode system.[43] A number of metal alloys were considered. Among them were orthodontic gold, which was rejected (perhaps wrongly) because of its copper content. Pure platinum proved too soft. A number of alloying elements were considered with platinum to harden it. Among them were rhodium, palladium, nickel, and iridium. Iridium was selected and was alloyed up to 10 percent, 20 percent, 30 percent, and 40 percent content. The higher percentages proved too brittle, and 10 percent was finally selected. The resulting filamentary wire was stronger than structural steel, but still would not survive the flexing fatigue of the body environment until it was wound into a spring coil structure. This lead met the need and along with the Swedish poly-ethylene leads became the industry standard for the first decade of pace-making, until displaced by the transvenous catheter in the late 1960s.

3. Spring Coil Endocardial Catheter Leads

The first permanent transvenous catheter was the Chardack/Medtronic (5816). Unsupported transvenous catheters are not stiff enough to be independently inserted (usually through the external jugular vein). Also, there is no way to manipulate the tip past obstructions such as the heart valves and into a desirable final position, deep in the apex of the ventricle. Therefore, a stylet is provided, having the distal end slightly bent. The stylet provides a stiffer structure to facilitate placement. Rotation of the stylet causes a rotary motion of the bent tip, facilitating manipulation of the electrode past interfering structures of the heart.

Platinum 10 percent iridium proved to be too weak to withstand insertion of the stylet. The coil turns separated, allowing the stylet to slip between turns and perforate the silicone sheath. A number of iron chromium cobalt alloys (304 and 316 stainless steel, Elgiloy and MP35) all proved strong enough and have seen extensive clinical use.

Originally the stylet was left in place, but it soon became evident that the monofilament straight stylet was subjected by heart motion to bending stresses greater than it could stand. When the stylet broke, all the bending stress on the whole adjacent lead area was concentrated at the break, very soon resulting in lead rupture.

Stainless steel is actually an industrial resistance wire, and stainless steel coil leads have a much higher resistance than platinum leads. This resistance can be markedly reduced by winding the coils with a number of parallel wires rather than a single wire. Such coils are termed double-pitch if two wires are used, or triple-pitch if three wires are used. If three wires are used, each wire will be one third as long because each wire supplies only one third of the coils. Thus, each wire has only one third the resistance of a single pitch coil. Since three such coils are connected in parallel, the resistance is reduced by another factor of three. Thus, a triple-pitch coil lead has only one ninth of the resistance of a comparable single-pitch coil lead.

Some leads, such as osteogenic or infection control leads, are located in areas of the body with much less motion; therefore, less bending stress is incurred. In such leads less strength may be satisfactory, and special materials (such as silver for silver ion germicidal control) may be needed. Table 4 shows the relative strengths of several platinum and silver metals.

Transvenous leads are subjected to large stresses and must be carefully mechanically designed if rupture is to be avoided. Stresses will concentrate at any abrupt change in diameter or any abrupt change of the mechanical strength of the structure. Thus, any change in diameter must be a gradual one, and any abrupt change in materials must be cushioned by supporting structures of silicone or other material. Figure 29 shows a coil lead structure where three different diameters of silicone rubber sheath are telescoped to reduce stresses at points of structure change. Insulating materials must be carefully chosen. Silicone rubber is a much-used material and is probably the most readily accepted by the body.

E. *The Electrode*

The electrode is the portion of the conducting structure which actually contacts the heart, or any other site which is to be driven or sensed. In some structures, such as spring-coil myocardial electrodes, strength and stress relief is very important. In other structures, such as endocardial catheter tips, little stress is seen, and material strength is not important. The electrode must not attack the body and it must not be attacked by it. This limits the metals that can be used to just a few possibilities. Platinum and its alloys are the most used. Stainless steel, Elgiloy, MP35 (Imploy), and titanium have seen some use.

Some newer, nonmetal materials have been suggested and used clinically. One example is an activated vitreous carbon structure reported by G. Richter[44] of Siemans in Europe. The present author has examined carbon materials but found them objectionably polarizable, as reported above by Richter.[45] However, the proprietary activation process used seems to have markedly alleviated this problem. One wishes that the process were not so proprietary so that one might evaluate the long-term prognosis of such an electrode with more confidence. With this electrode, as with other new advances, some years of experience will probably be required to justify a departure from the many highly reliable and highly satisfactory electrode types now available.

1. Myocardial Electrodes

Early myocardial electrodes advanced from the simple wires of C. Walton Lillehei et al.,[46] to the bipolar pins of Samuel Hunter et al.,[47] to the spring coil structures of William Chardack,[48] and to the screw-in structures of today. Probably not more than 10 percent of new implants today use the myocardial approach, although it is the method of choice if the chest must be opened for other reasons. We have previously mentioned that surgical block in a child is 100 percent fatal within one year without a pacemaker if acute block lasts more than three weeks. The same type of cardiac arrest occurs in many heart transplant patients who characteristically have two sinus nodes, one their own and one from the donor heart. It has been suggested that perhaps every heart transplant patient should also receive a pacemaker at transplant. In such a case, myocardial electrodes would be a preferred choice.

It was observed with early Hunter Roth electrodes that those with imperfectly polished pins tended to seat better in the myocardium. Highly polished pins tended to move more, creating a fluid pocket which resulted in a much higher threshold. Thus, roughened or screen surfaces would seem to be more quickly and more securely fixed in the heart. This will be discussed in more detail under porous electrodes.

2. Endocardial Electrodes

Endocardial electrodes generally become encased in a collagenous layer of tissue on the endocardium. They are therefore not subject to the severe shear stresses seen by myocardial electrodes which may pass through several layers of muscle, each contracting in a different plane. Pure platinum has adequate strength for such an application and is commonly used.

Stainless steel, Elgiloy, and MP35 also see some use, but much more care must be taken with surface finish. Microcracks in the surface can lead to crevice corrosion. The valley of the crack becomes positively charged with respect to the surface, and anodic corrosion begins. This corrosion progresses, deepening the crack until failure occurs. A typical example from the orthopedic field is the case of a wide-flange bone screw against a bone plate. Corrosion begins at the juncture of the pin and the plate, under the flange, and the area becomes oxygen-starved. For lack of oxygen, chloride corrosion begins which leads to the failure. If the surface were perfectly smooth, a copious supply of oxygen from the body would maintain the protective oxide coating, and no corrosion would take place.

Stainless steel itself is stainless only because of this tough oxide coating. Without it, stainless steel corrodes easily. Actually, such corrosion is rarely seen on stainless steel stimulating cathodes because they are highly polished and they are "cathodically protected" by the stimulating pulse. Another example from another field is the case of an iron pipe crossing under a roadbed whose base is slag or cinders, both of which are acid. The section of pipe under the road corrodes much sooner than that passing through near-neutral farm soil. It is common practice to bury a piece of scrap iron near the pipe and to connect a battery to them so as to drive the scrap iron positive and the pipe negative. The scrap iron becomes a "sacrificial anode" and corrodes readily, but the

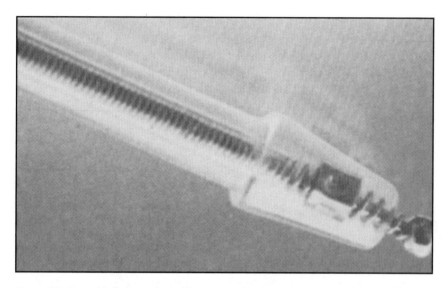

Figure 23. Typical ball-point electrode (Cordis). The ball is 1 mmD, and the area is 8 mm^2.

pipe, being "cathodically protected," is spared. Every few years the piece of scrap iron and the battery must be replaced. A more satisfactory chemical solution is to use crushed limestone (which is not acidic) for the roadbed.

Some endocardial electrodes are so connected that a short-circuit or DC leakage in the output capacitor will drive a positive current through the electrode. This results in necrosis (tissue death), electrode corrosion, and gas generation.

These same problems apply to the counter electrode, which is usually the metal plate on the side of the pulse generator. This electrode is an anode and therefore particularly subject to corrosion. The juncture of the epoxy insulation and the plate is a natural site for oxygen deprivation and crevice corrosion. Some degree of such corrosion can sometimes be seen at this juncture in unipolar pulse generators with stainless steel plates that have been in service for many years. Such corrosion is not seen with titanium plates, or with the more modern hermetically sealed metal-encased pacemakers, particularly those with titanium cases.

3. Parsonnet Differential Current Density Electrode

Anthony Mauro[49] originally suggested an electrode structure that had a large area of platinum electrode exposed to body electrolyte in a closed, insulated cavity. The cavity made electrical contact to body tissue through a small hole through the insulated wall. This resulted in minimal polarization losses at the metal surface due to the large area, but maximum current density at the stimulation site because of the small size of the hole. Losses at the hole would be only those due to the ohmic drop in the fluid and any liquid junction potentials that might develop. Victor Parsonnet[50] developed this idea into a clinical electrode, which saw successful use in his hands.

The concept did not find universal acceptance since it was necessary to locate the small hole opening adjacent to a viable stimulation side. Results in all hands were not consistent. Nevertheless, this concept did find use in a modified form as the "porous" electrode to be discussed below.

4. Ball-Point Electrode

Electrodes such as the older large-area platinum electrodes (Figure 4) had such a low impedance that battery current was sometimes excessive. Subsequent endocardial electrode designs were usually much smaller. One of the smallest of the contemporary electrodes was no larger than the tip of a ball-point pen. Thus it has commonly become known as the "ball-point" electrode.[51] Its electrode area is only 8 mm^2 compared to the 80 mm^2 area of the older Medtronic/Chardack 5816 (Figure 23).

Werner Irnich[52] and others have shown that smaller electrodes produce a higher current density at the stimulation site and are therefore generally more efficient. There is a limit, however, as to how small an electrode can be without getting into an area of diminishing returns. If an electrode is too big, it will have a low current density and dissipate its energy too widely. However, results with it will be very consistent. If the electrode is too small, it may well be far from a viable stimulation site and will have a markedly higher impedance, both to stimulating currents and to sensing voltages in the case of demand pacemakers. Irnich et al.[53] found the optimum electrode size to be a diameter approximately that of the distance from the electrode to the nearest viable stimulation site. We also find this to be true (see Figure 3).

Thus, there are advantages to small electrodes but there may be serious disadvantages to having them too small. Consistency of stimulation threshold from one patient to the next will not be as good for the very small structures. Also, the higher impedance must be taken into account in pulse generator design, both in making enough driving voltage available to overcome the higher impedance of the electrode and in providing a very high input impedance in the pulse generator sensing

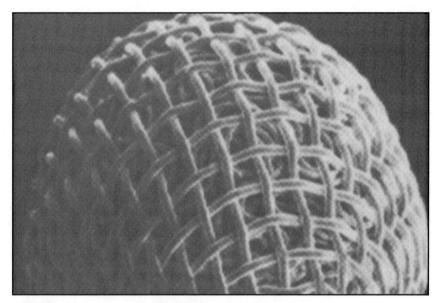

Figure 24. Amundson/CPI porous electrode.

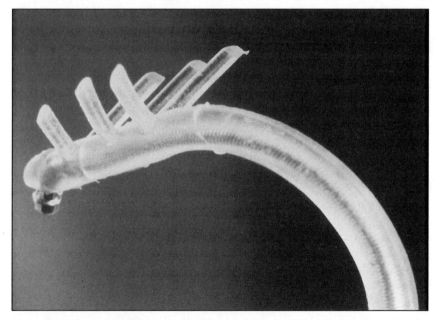

Figure 25. "J" type atrial electrode (Medtronic 6991). The "J" structure, along with the silicone rubber tines, tends to support the structure in the atrium. The tines are trimmed at implant to whatever length is felt to be optimum.

amplifier so that the higher impedance of the small electrode will not result in excessive voltage loss in the sensed R wave.

5. Amundson Porous Electrode

From previous discussions it is clear that the ideal electrode would have a large area of metal/electrolyte interface, but a small cross-sectional area of current delivery. The porous electrode of D. Amundson[54] accomplished this in a unique way. A hemispherical platinum screen at the electrode tip encloses a ball of compacted platinum iridium wire fibers of 20 μm diameter. The combined surface areas of the two structures add up to a much larger surface than would be attainable with an electrode of conventional structure.

Another advantage of this structure is the rapid ingrowth of tissue into the screen. Fixation seemed to be accomplished very soon after placement, minimizing the possibility of early displacement due to the mechanical trauma that occurs in some cases. Also, the stimulation threshold of mature (six-month) electrodes seemed to rise to a lesser degree than that of more conventional structures (Figure 24).

Successful clinical use of this electrode has been reported by N. Berman and D. Lipton[55] of Toronto and others.

Another interesting approach to a porous structure has been reported by S. Miller of Cordis.[56] A solid metal substrate is coated with a metal powder which is sintered into the substrate at high temperatures in a reducing atmosphere. This method is adapted from one used to accelerate the fixation of orthopedic prostheses to surrounding bone. McGregor et al. report success with this electrode as an atrial electrode in experimental animals.[57]

6. Atrial Electrodes

To be truly "physiological," a pacemaker should pick up the P wave on the atrium, amplify and delay the sensed signal, and deliver it to the ventricle as a processed R wave about a tenth of a second later than the P wave. Some early pacemaking systems did exactly this and were pronounced more physiological. Two electrodes were required, one on the atrium and one on the ventricle, both placed via a thoracotomy. They never achieved as much as 1 percent of the total pacemaker market because of difficulties with the atrial electrode. The P wave is only a fraction of the amplitude of the R wave, and its source is so located as to make it very difficult to mechanically secure an electrode in its vicinity. Also, the much greater amplitude of the R wave means that some means of frequency discrimination or spatial discrimination must be employed.

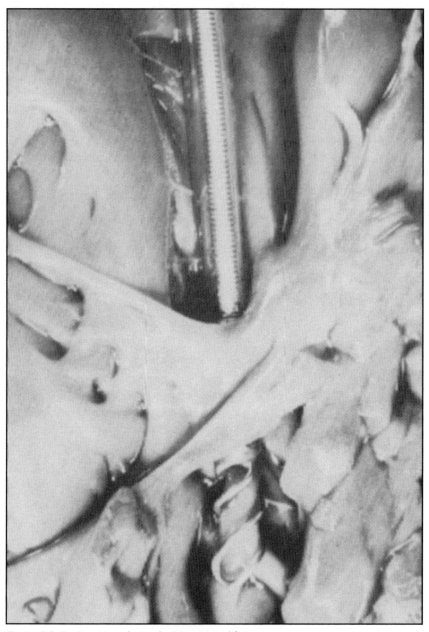

Figure 26. Fixation type electrode (Vitatron Helifix).

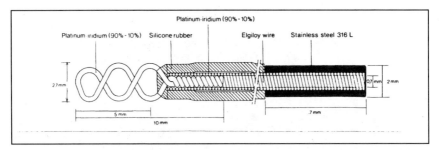

Figure 27. "Helifix" electrode (Vitatron Helifix). The helical coils tend to wind into the trabeculae to lock the electrode in place.

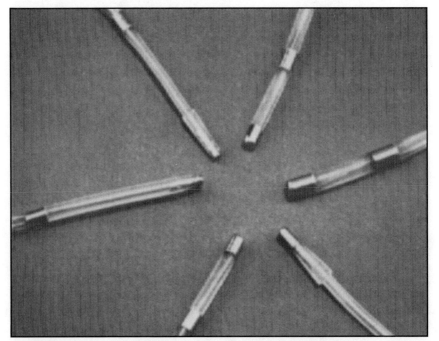

Figure 28. Transvenous endocardial catheter electrodes (Medtronic). Fixation of some of these electrodes is facilitated by the silicone rubber flange around the tip.

When a synchronous pacing system failed, the reason was usually related to the atrial electrode.

Some more recent systems have circumvented this problem by using atrial electrodes which are only used to drive the atrium and are not required to sense. This is a help, but even so, the atrial electrode is still a limiting factor.

In early systems, it was not possible to place the atrial electrode via

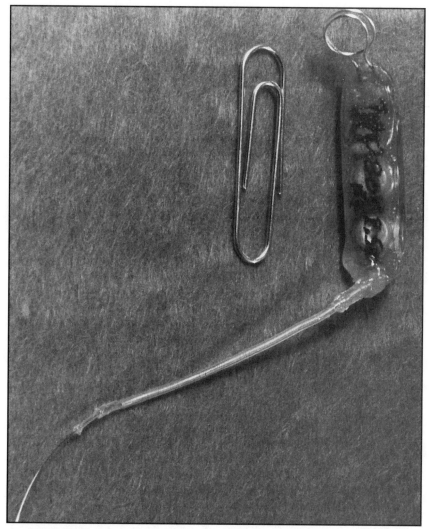

Figure 29. Osteogenic stimulator with an Ag 10% Pd spring coil structure (made by the author).

the transvenous route. A thoracotomy was required. More recently, two endocardial approaches have been used. In one, the atrial electrode is formed into a "J" shaped structure which supports itself against the walls of the atrium (Figure 25). In one case, silicone rubber tines were added to assist in the fixation (Medtronic 6991).

Another approach is to position an electrode in the coronary sinus. Even though this approach is from the ventricle, a properly positioned electrode will be quite near the source of atrial signals and can success-fully discriminate them from the ventricular R wave. Additional fixation means are sometimes employed. S. Joseph and J. White[58] have reported successful use of the Vitatron "Helifix" electrode in the coronary sinus. G. Wilson et al.[59] have used the Cordis porous electrode as an atrial elec-trode in the coronary sinus.

Each international meeting predicts extensive use of atrial pace-making. The limiting factor still is the need for two electrodes (double trouble) and the higher probability of poor reliability of function of the atrial electrode.

7. Fixation-Type Electrodes

Early and late displacement of endocardial catheter electrodes have accounted for about a 10 percent failure of pacing. Since the advent of the lithium battery, nearly all surgical interventions necessitated for pacemaker repair have been electrode-related. Thus, the profession has long sought some means to decrease the incidence of early and late elec-trode displacement. We have already discussed the screw-in myocardial electrode, which was one step in this direction.

European efforts have been directed toward tined structures with barbs which can be propelled outward from the seated electrode, pinning it in place. Werner Irnich[60] proposed a two-tine structure that was man-ufactured by Biotronik (Model IG 65-1). A similar structure with four nylon bristles as tines was manufactured by Vitatron (Model MIP 2000). Another approach, again by Vitatron (Helifix), utilized a helical electrode structure designed to be caught up in the trabeculae of the heart, fixing the electrode in position. (See Figures 26 and 27.)

American efforts were more in the direction of silicone rubber flanges which would catch on the trabeculae when forced through them (Figure 28). The problem has been to provide enough fixation so that the electrode would not displace, but not so much fixation that the heart wall was damaged or penetrated.

Electrode Structures for Osteogenesis and Infection Control

Devices for osteogenesis and infection control are generally DC devices operating with output currents between 1 and 80 µA. Since this is still a developing field, the stimulation parameters remain somewhat contro-versial. C. Brighton et al.[61] have confined themselves to external stimu-lators with four acute percutaneous monofilament stainless steel cathodes, each delivering 20 µA for a total of 80 µA. Stimulation is continued for eight to twelve weeks, after which the electrodes are withdrawn.

In our own work in infection control in plants and animals,[62] we have used lower currents, generally below 10 µA, to corrode a silver wire. The resulting silver ion environment has proved germicidal to a number of plant and animal bacteria and to plant viroids. Joseph Spadero et al.[63] have used this same technique to kill floating tumor cells of the mouse ascites variety.

Totally implantable osteogenic stimulators were manufactured by Teletronic Pty. Ltd. in Australia. They generally used a 20 µA DC current on a stainless steel cathode with a titanium anode.

In our own work with total implants, we have used a single pitch, spring coil electrode structure of about 5 cm in length, continuing in a monofilament structure another 5 cm. The spring coil is encased in a silicone sheath. Three different thicknesses of silicone sheath are used to alleviate any strains that might exist at the stimulator wall and at the end of the coil. Figure 29 shows the stimulator with its electrode.

We have built such electrodes from pure silver, silver with 10 percent palladium, pure platinum, and platinum 10 percent iridium. We have a philosophical bias against stainless steel because it is not really stainless.

NOTES

1. C. Beck, W. Pritchard, and H. Feil, "Ventricular Fibrillation of Long Duration Abolished By Electrical Shock." *Journal of the American Medical Association* 135 (1947): 985.

2. P. Zoll, "Resuscitation of the Heart in Ventricular Stand-still By External Electric Stimulation." *New England Journal of Medicine* 247 (1952): 768.

3. W. Greatbatch and W. Chardack, "A Transistorized Implantable Pacemaker, etc." *Proc. NEREM*, Boston 1 (1959): 8.

4. W. Chardack, E. Gage, and W. Greatbatch, "A Transistorized, Self-contained, Implantable Pacemaker for the Long-term Correction of Complete Heart Block." *Surgery* 18, no. 4 (1960): 643.

5. I. Yasuda, "On the Piezoelectric Effect of Bone." *J. Physiol. Soc.*, Japan 10 (1957): 1158.

6. C. Brighton, Z. Friedenberg, E. Mitchell, and R. Booth, "Treatment of Non-union with Constant Direct Current." *Clin. Orthop.* 124 (1977): 106.

7. R. Becker and J. Spadero, "Treatment of Orthopedic Infections with Electrically Generated Silver Ions." *J. Bone Jt. Surg.* 60A, no. 7 (1978): 871.

8. J. Spadero, T. Berger, S. Barranco, S. Chapin, and R. Becker, "Antibacterial Effects of Silver Electrodes with Weak Direct Current." *Antimicrob. Agents Chemother.* 6, no. 5 (1974): 637.

9. W. Greatbatch, B. Piersma, F. Shannon, and S. Calhoon, "Polarization

Phenomena Relating to Physiological Electrodes." *Ann. N. Y. Acad. Sci.* 167, no. 2 (1969): 722.

10. S. Brummer and M. Turner, "Electrical Stimulation with Pt Electrodes." BME 24, *IEEE Trans. Biomed. Eng.* 5 (1977): 436.

11. B. Piersma, F. Shannon, S. Calhoon, and W. Greatbatch, "Electrochemical Polarization of Physiological Electrodes, etc." "Electrochemical Bioscience and Bioengineering," *Proc. Electrochem. Soc.*, Chicago (1974): 133.

12. D. Salkin, ed., "Electrochemical Bioscience and Bioengineering." *Trans. Electrochemical Society*, Chicago, spring 1973.

13. W. Nernst, *Z. Phys. Chem.* 4 (1889): 129.

14. A. Kahn and W. Greatbatch, "Physiological Electrodes." In *Medical Engineering 79*, edited by C. Ray. (Chicago: Year Book Medical Publishing, 1973), 1073.

15. K. Cole, "Alternating Current Conductance and Direct Current Excitation of a Nerve." *Science* 79 (1934): 164.

16. P. Mansfield, "Myocardial Stimulation: The Electrochemistry of Electrode-tissue Coupling." *Am. J. Physiol.* 212, no. 6 (1967): 1475.

17. J. Weinman and J. Mahler, "An Analysis of Electrical Properties of Metal Electrodes." *Med. Electron. Biol. Eng.* 2 (1964): 265.

18. W. Greatbatch et al., "Polarization Phenomena Relating to Physiological Electrodes," 722.

19. Ibid.

20. S. Brummer and M. Turner, "Electrical Stimulation with Pt Electrodes," 436.

21. B. Piersma et al., "Electrochemical Polarization of Physiological Electrodes, etc.," 133.

22. T. Warner, S. Schuldiner, and B. Piersma, "On the Activity of Platinum Catalysts in Solution." *J. Electrochem. Soc.* 114 (1967): 1120.

23. B. Piersma et al., "Electrochemical Polarization of Physiological Electrodes, etc.," 133.

24. Ibid.

25. R. Becker and J. Spadero, "Treatment of Orthopedic Infection"; J. Spadero et al., "Antibacterial Effects of Silver Electrodes"; W. Greatbatch, *Proc. XI Intl. Conf. Med. Biol. Eng.*, Jerusalem, 1979.

26. C. Hall and J. Hackerman, *J. Phys. Chem.* 57 (1971): 262.

27. B. Piersma, S. Calhoon, and W. Greatbatch, "Some Comparisons of Pt and Ti Physiological Electrolytes." *Proc. Electrochem. Soc.*, Chicago, spring 1973: 133.

28. J. Davies and E. Sowton, "Electrical Threshold of the Human Heart." *Br. Heart J.* 28 (1966): 231.

29. W. Greatbatch, "Energy Losses in Cardiac Electrodes as a Function of Pulse Duration." Unpublished material, 1966.

30. K. Cole, "Alternating Current Conductance and Direct Current Excitation of a Nerve," 164.

31. S. Hunter, N. Roth, D. Bernardez, and J. Noble, "A Bipolar Myocardial Electrode for Complete Heart Block." *Lancet* 79 (1959): 506.

32. C. Lillehei, A. Gott, P. Hodges, D. Long, and E. Bakken, "Transistorized

Pacemaker for Treatment of Complete Heart Block." *Journal of the American Medical Association* 172 (1960): 2006.

33. Ibid.

34. Ibid.

35. S. Hunter et al., "A Bipolar Myocardial Electrode for Complete Heart Block," 506.

36. W. Greatbatch and W. Chardack, "A Transistorized Implantable Pacemaker, etc.," 8.

37. W. Chardack, E. Gage, and W. Greatbatch, "A Transistorized, Self-contained, Implantable Pacemaker for the Long-term Correction of Complete Heart Block," 643.

38. W. Chardack, "A Myocardial Electrode for Long-term Pacemaker, III." *Ann. N.Y. Acad. Sci.* 3 (1964): 893.

39. H. Lagergren, "How It Happened: My Recollection of Early Pacing." *PACE* 1 (1978): 140.

40. S. Furman and J. Schwedel, "Intracardiac Pacemaker for Stokes-Adams Seizures." *New England Journal of Medicine* 261 (1959): 943.

41. W. Chardack, "A Myocardial Electrode for Long-term Pacemaker, III," 893.

42. Ibid.

43. Ibid.

44. G. Richter, E. Weidlich, F. Sturm, E. David, G. Brandt, H. Elmqvist, and A. Thoren, "Nonpolarizable Vitreous Carbon Pacing Electrodes." *Proc. VI World Pacing Symp.*, Montreal, 29 (1979): 13.

45. Ibid.

46. C. Lillehei et al., "Transistorized Pacemaker for Treatment of Complete Heart Block," 2006.

47. S. Hunter et al., "A Bipolar Myocardial Electrode for Complete Heart Block," 506.

48. W. Chardack, "A Myocardial Electrode for Long-term Pacemaker, III," 893.

49. A. Mauro, "Capacity Electrode for Chronic Stimulation." *Science* 132 (1960): 356.

50. V. Parsonnet, I. Zucker, L. Gilbert, G. Lewine, G. Myers, and R. Avery, "Clinical Use of a New Transvenous Electrode." *Ann. N.Y. Acad. Sci.* 167, no. 2 (1969): 756.

51. S. Furman, P. Hurzeler, and R. Mehra, "Cardiac Pacing and Pacemakers. IV. Threshold of Cardiac Stimulation." *Am. Heart J.* 94 (1977): 115.

52. W. Bleifeld, W. Irnich, and S. Effert, "A New Transvenous Electrode with Myocardial Fixation." *Proc. IX Int. Conf. Med. Biol. Eng.*, Melbourne, 10, no. 4 (1971): 76.

53. Ibid.

54. D. Amundsen, W. McArthur, and M. Mosharrafa, "A New Porous Electrode for Endocardial Stimulation." *PACE* 2, no. 1 (1979): 40.

55. N. Berman and D. Lipton, "Early Clinical Experience with a Porous Tip Electrode." *PACE* 2, no. 5 (1979): A86.

56. G. Wilson, D. MacGregor, J. Bobyn, W. Lixfield, R. Pilliar, S. Miller, and

M. Silver, "Tissue Response to Porous-surfaced Electrodes." *Proc. VI World Pacing Symp.*, Montreal, 29 (1979): 12.

57. Ibid.

58. S. Joseph and J. White, "Permanent Atrial Pacing: Functional Characteristics of Coronary Sinus and Right Atrial Appendage Electrodes." *Proc. VI World Pacing Symp.*, Montreal, 29 (1979): 6.

59. G. Wilson et al., "Tissue Response to Porous-surfaced Electrodes," 12.

60. W. Bleifeld, W. Irnich, and S. Effert, "A New Transvenous Electrode with Myocardial Fixation," 76.

61. C. Brighton et al., "Treatment of Non-union with Constant Direct Current," 106.

62. W. Greatbatch, *Proc. XI Int. Conf. Med. Biol. Eng.*

63. J. Spadero, T. Berger, S. Barranco, S. Chapin, and R. Becker, "Antibacterial Effects of Silver Electrodes with Weak Direct Current." *Antimicrob. Agents Chemother.* 6, no. 5 (1974): 637.

FOR FURTHER READING

Greatbatch, W. "Polarization Phenomena Relating to Physiological Electrodes." *Ann. N. Y. Acad. Sci.* 167 (1969): 2.

Lewin, G., G. Meyers, and V. Parsonnet, "Differential Current Density Electrodes for Pacemakers." *Proc. 19th Annu. Conf. Eng. Med. Biol.* 8 (1966): 165.

Nathan, D., S. Center, C. Wu, and W. Keller, "An Implantable Synchronous Pacemaker for the Long-term Correction of Complete Heart Block." *Am. J. Cardiol.*, 11 (1963): 362.

Schwann, H., C. Kay, and T. Bothwell, "Electrical Resistivity of Body Tissues at Low Frequencies." *Proc. Fed. Biol. Soc.* 13 (1954): 1.

4

POWER SOURCES

INTRODUCTION*

The introduction of the lithium battery in 1971[1] was a real cultural shock to the pacemaker manufacturers. It did represent a large step toward the "lifetime pacemaker," but necessitated a radical change in pacemaker design philosophy which few manufacturers were willing to accept. The advent of hermetic sealing probably precluded the use of multicell batteries, and the resulting use of a single-cell battery made it necessary to include a voltage multiplier in the pacemaker circuit. Worse yet, pacemaker circuit designers had been used to designing for the end-of-life impedance of the zinc mercury cell of about ten ohms. They had to revise their thinking to accommodate the end-of-life impedance of the lithium iodine cell of as much as 50,000 ohms. We anticipated extreme reluctance on their part to do this and responded by building some prototype lithium demonstration pacemakers. Naturally, the larger manufacturers were the most reluctant to change. Medtronic would not change until we agreed (against our will) to build them a two-cell battery, which went successfully into their Xyrel model. Cordis never went to a single-cell battery, in spite of our incessant prodding. I attribute much of their subsequent decline to their reluctance to change. Eventually the advantages of the lithium iodine design became universally recognized, and by 1990 all of the world's pacemakers used it.

Nearly all of the early implantable pacemakers were powered by

---

*Please refer to the appendix for this chapter at the back of this book for more information.

119

zinc mercury batteries. However, by 1970 the average life of the pulse generator was only two years, with about 80 percent of the removals necessitated by failed batteries. It was clear that the power source was the principal mode of failure and that no significant improvement could be expected until this problem was solved. Yet, we should not be overcritical of these early mercury batteries. Even with all their problems, they made pacemaking possible and they continued to dominate the field for fifteen years.

In 1968, we began a search for an improved power source. We followed two paths. One led through halide cathodes, all using lithium as an anode. The other led through nuclear batteries, most using plutonium[238] (Pu) as an alpha particle emitting heat generator. We also considered rechargeable batteries and biological power sources, but rejected both for reasons we will discuss later.

Our lithium experiments began with cathodes of nickel sulphide, that we could not seal. We then evaluated sulphur dioxide cathodes (which required pressurization at three atmospheres). We could not control the reactions and several cells burst, contaminating our warm-rooms. We examined thionyl chloride, but were concerned about the instability of the anode interface coating. We finally settled on an iodine cathode, after the teachings of James Moser and Alan Schneider,[2] and successfully introduced the first lithium cells into clinical usage.[3]

Our nuclear experiments, in collaboration with Hittman Corp. of Columbia, Maryland, were confined to the plutonium[238] isotope and resulted in a clinically satisfactory cell.[4] This cell saw some limited clinical use in American Optical Corp. and Cordis Corp. pacemakers. In a parallel program, Medtronic, using French plutonium[238] batteries with a bismuth telluride thermopile, manufactured a number of successful nuclear pacemakers, many of which are still in use. However, the total number of nuclear pacemakers of all kinds never approached 1 percent of the total of pacemakers implanted annually, largely because of the regulatory problems associated with control of the critical nuclear fuel. We know of no nuclear pacemakers being manufactured in 2000.

We decided in 1971 to divert our entire effort to the lithium iodine cell and terminated our work on nuclear batteries. By 1980, lithium batteries powered over 95 percent of the world's pacemaker production. Most of these were lithium iodine types and were available from a number of pacemaker manufacturers.

With the advent of more sophisticated pacemaker designs, the need for additional current capability began to push the design limits of the lithium iodine system to uncomfortable margins. New pacemaker functional requirements such as implanted telemetry, arrythmia control, implantable defibrillation, and programmed trains of pulses, all required a higher current capability of the battery, although not necessarily requiring a greater total energy capability. Having anticipated this need, we had begun studying other lithium systems in the mid-1970s, most of which used a liquid electrolyte. We actually built a few lithium bromine batteries[5] which looked promising, but proved unreproducible, at least to the consistency required for good production. This finally evolved into a lithium-chlorine-bromine complex cell,[6] quite different from the original cell, but with more consistent properties. Following this was a lithium sulphuryl chloride cell,[7] which could operate at 150°C, and another solid lithium silver vanadium oxide cell.[8] The latter two can be made autoclavable.

With autoclavable batteries, we were in a position of being able to promote the concept of totally autoclavable implantable devices. We believed this to be a concept whose time had come. Until then, pacemaker batteries had never been autoclavable. In the year 2000, we still feel autoclavable pacemakers make good sense, but the profession has not gone in that direction.

We saw pacemakers and pacemaker power sources as being on the threshold of another giant leap forward with full microprocessor computing capability to handle not only selectable stimulation modes, but many therapeutic corrective modes. With the emerging array of implantable sensors, we could perhaps implement many previously unavailable diagnostic modes. An accumulative, interrogable, storage memory would cover the lifetime of the pulse generator itself. New

---

THE WAY IT WAS

The conventional flashlight battery (Le Clanche cell) required about seventy years to emerge from the laboratory into full production. In contrast, the Ruben Mallory cell ("RM" series) was immediately classified by the U.S. government and required only one year to go from laboratory prototype to a production level of a million per day. It was not until two years after WW II ended that the details of this revolutionary development appeared in the technical literature.[9]

* * *

We learned of this cell in 1958 through the aggressive sales work of Gordon Kaye. Through his efforts and those of Joseph D'Alfonso and Robert Mainzer, we had their watch batteries in our pacemakers before they ever got them into their watches.

power sources would be needed, but the technology was available and the future looked bright.

ZINC MERCURY BATTERIES

Prior to World War II the only primary battery in general use was the carbon manganese dioxide Le Clanche cell. World War II "walkie-talkies" required a much better power source, and Dr. Samuel Ruben developed the zinc mercury system which met the need.[10] His device was commercialized by the Mallory Company, and hundreds of millions of Ruben-Mallory zinc mercury batteries were made during the next four decades.

The Ruben Mallory cell provided greater energy density and better reliability than previous systems, but was subject to significant internal self-discharge which meant a rather short shelf life, particularly at body temperature. In 1958–60 Mallory modified the zinc mercury cell for longer shelf life at low current rates. The market objective was electronic

THE WAY IT WAS

An early epoxy encapsulated pulse generator (Medtronic Model 5850) was returned to the company with a failed battery. The pacemaker had failed, then recovered function again and was pacing the patient when removed. Upon examination we found a large hard epoxy bubble on one side. We couldn't understand how the bubble got there. It was brittle and shattered when we pressed it. We finally analyzed the sequence of events as follows: 1) A cell had shorted, releasing considerable hydrogen gas. Pressure built up until the neoprene seal vented and released the gas, and some sodium hydroxide, into the outer shell of the cell. 2) Pressure built up until it broke the weld between the two battery caps, opening up the battery string and causing the pacemaker to fail. 3) The hydrogen and sodium hydroxide then vented into the epoxy encapsulation. The sodium hydroxide softened the epoxy and the hydrogen gas blew up the bubble. 4) The defective cell discharged itself, pressure dropped, and the battery caps remade contact, causing the pacemaker to resume function, but with one less cell in the ten-cell string. 5) The sodium hydroxide and hydrogen diffused innocuously out into the body, leaving the epoxy bubble to harden up into a brittle, but intact, form. A real study in battery biochemistry!

wrist watches. The potassium hydroxide electrolyte was replaced by less active sodium hydroxide. A small amount of manganese dioxide was added to delay the onset of internal self-discharge until after the cell was in use. This resulted in a slightly higher voltage (1.5v) during the first 10 percent of life. Thus, an open-circuit voltage measurement of 1.5v insured a new cell. After the initial plateau had burned off, the cell dropped to its 1.345v normal voltage which it held, within millivolts, until end-of-life.

Later developments included the addition of some silver into the mix to amalgamate with the liquid mercury which was a byproduct of the battery reaction. All these modifications helped, but by 1970 the average pace-

THE WAY IT WAS

In the 1960s we made many trips to Mallory at Tarrytown, New York, trying to track down our battery problems. I'm afraid we did quite a bit of desk pounding. D'Alfonso used to gather his experts around the table and add up their years of employment with Mallory. He then expounded on the power of the 200 years of accumulated battery experience he was bringing to bear on our problem. It was a very impressive show but still didn't fix the battery.

During one visit I saw an X-ray of a flashlight battery that had been returned from England. All the internal structure was clearly apparent. I asked if a similar X-ray of a mercury battery might not reveal the degree of discharge. The Mallory people said no, that discharge produced no chemical changes that an X-ray could pick up.

I didn't quite believe that and when I got home, I discharged several groups of cells down to 90 percent, 80 percent, and 50 percent capacity. I then took them to the Symington Wayne Company that manufactured railroad car wheels in nearby Depew, New York. Among their quality control equipment was a giant X-ray machine that they used to detect hairline cracks in the wheel castings. Mr. Suckow was extremely cooperative and X-rayed my cells for me.

Analysis of the film proved that we could easily identify as little as 5 percent discharge with about a ±5 percent accuracy. We published our results[11] and it was not long before our X-ray analysis method became pretty much the standard throughout the pacemaker industry. There is nothing more satisfying than doing something that the experts say you can't do.

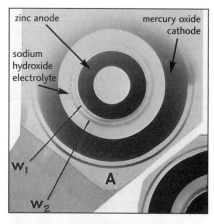

zinc anode

mercury oxide cathode

sodium hydroxide electrolyte

w_1

w_2

A

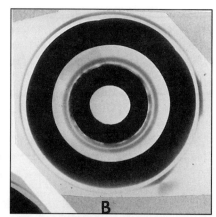

B

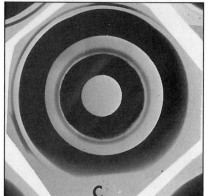

C

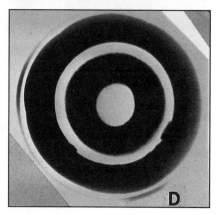

D

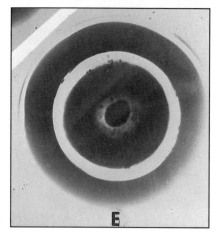

E

X-Ray Evaluation of Zinc-Mercury Cell Rundown:

A. New cell. Note the clear, sharp outlines. Note case discontinuities w_1, w_2 which serve as gauge marks of cell discharge.

B. 10 percent discharged. Note that the zinc anode cylinder now has a fuzzy outline.

C. 30 percent discharged. Ring w_1 is encompassed.

D. 50 percent discharged. Both w_1 and w_2 rings are now encompassed.

E. Over 80 percent discharged. The inter-electrode electrolyte area is much reduced and globules of liquid mercury obscure the center anode hole.

maker was being removed and replaced in less than two years[12] with about 80 percent of these being explanted because of failure of the battery.

The corrosive liquid electrolyte (sodium hydroxide) still led to long-term degradation of the separator and the high pressure of hydrogen gas (typically 300 psig) eliminated the possibility of hermetically sealing the cell. Incomplete utilization of the evolved mercury by the silver additive led to occasional failure due to mercury dendrites bridging anode and cathode. Along with the evolved hydrogen gas, some sodium hydroxide electrolyte was also exuded. Both dissipated innocuously through the epoxy encapsulation into the body but left us with some concern and a few untoward effects.

In desperation we sought for some means of nondestructively analyzing zinc mercury cells. The military also had the same problem. They attacked it by periodically sampling warehouse lots of stored batteries and running the sample down to exhaustion. If and when the samples showed less than acceptable capacity, the whole warehouse lot was removed from inventory.

We developed a method of X-ray analysis that proved quite effective in identifying as little as a 5 percent discharge by radiologically visualizing the diffusion of reaction by-products away from the cathode and the anode.

Our X-ray system soon came to be universally used to evaluate pacemaker pulse generators and/or their batteries. It was not uncommon to store completed pacemakers for thirty days at 37°C before shipment. Just prior to shipment the whole package was X-rayed. A satisfactory radiograph demonstrated that a) each cell had been satisfactorily man-

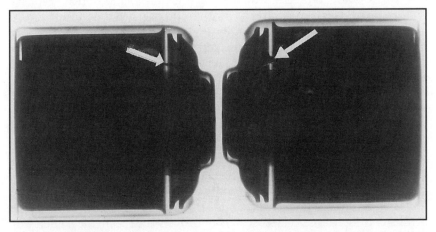

X-ray view of older RM-1 zinc-mercury pacemaker cells which failed due to growth of mercury dendrites. (Note the white arrows.)

ufactured; b) that it had not been accidentally shorted during pulse generator manufacture; c) that the pulse generator had functioned normally at 37°C for thirty days without visible battery degradation; and d) that all the necessary tools and hardware accessories were indeed included inside the sealed package.

An alternate zinc-mercury design by Le Clanche (Switzerland) gave some hope of overcoming various problems inherent in this system. The Le Clanche version used the original potassium hydroxide electrolyte, but used a planar rather than a cylindrical structure. As many as five layers of separators were used. Unfortunately, the measures taken by Le Clanche only delayed the inevitable breakdown. Later versions of this cell, as well as later comparable Mallory cells, seemed to indicate improved longevity, but by this time the trend to lithium had begun and no more zinc mercury cells were used in pacemakers.

THE SEARCH FOR A NEW POWER SOURCE

We had originally predicted a probable battery life of five years from the data supplied to us by the battery manufacturer.[13] However, by 1970 we were getting only two years. Several mechanisms contributed to the failure, most of them fundamental to the chemistry of the cell. The electrolyte is sodium hydroxide, which is very corrosive. The separator is one or more layers of webril, an organic material that is not particularly inert, which means it is subject to corrosion under the right conditions. Zinc oxide tends to migrate through the cell, forming conductive paths that drain the cell. As we previously mentioned, evolved hydrogen gas rises to pressures as high as 300 psig but then innocuously vents through the neoprene seal. By 1970 the zinc mercury battery was limiting the lifespan of the pacemaker. It was clear that little improvement could be expected in pacemaker performance until we could find a more reliable power source.

Many of us gave at least some consideration to every means of power generation or power storage that we could imagine. This included primary chemical batteries of all sorts, nuclear batteries, rechargeable batteries, and the separation of the system with the power pack being outside the body, transmitting pulses of energy to a passive implanted receiver. (Abrams in England, along with the Lucas automotive company, actually built and used a number of such units clinically, considerably before us, and with a better reliability than our early mercury-powered units.) Parsonnet considered piezo-electric bars to convert the mechanical energy of the beating heart into stored power. He also used a self-winding watch escapement. At least a half-dozen investigators considered making electricity electrochemically from the body's own chemistry.

BIOLOGICAL BATTERIES

The human body is a complex chemical system that contains many of the chemicals necessary for electrochemical production of electricity in a battery-like fashion. Many investigators have been attracted to this concept. P. Racine,[14] O. Roy,[15] M. Chaldach,[16] and others have considered biogalvanic cells. Gerald Cywinski[17] carried such a cell to three years of successful animal use. Others have considered fuel cell reactions utilizing oxygen from arterial blood and hydrogen from body proteins. Due to their marginal performance, no biological battery has yet seen any clinical use to date, and we consider this a dead issue as far as any practical pacemakers are concerned.

RECHARGEABLE BATTERIES

The concept of a small pacemaker battery, periodically rechargeable from an external source, is philosophically very attractive, but two questions must be answered: 1) Is the lifetime of the battery as good, with recharging, as the lifetime of a comparable primary cell, without recharging? 2) Is it medically acceptable to both physician and patient to give the patient control of the recharging function? The answer to *both* questions must be yes if the rechargeable system is to be acceptable. Furman recommended against the concept.[18] My good friend Alfred Mann and his Pacesetters company built and marketed several thousand such rechargeable pacemakers.

Senning's first implant in 1958 used a rechargeable nickel-cadmium cell. This system proved unsatisfactory[19] and it was soon abandoned. Since that time, papers have periodically appeared purporting to solve the problems inherent in this approach, but no rechargeable system has yet conclusively provided a sufficiently positive answer to the above two questions, and the rechargeable battery has never achieved 1 percent of the pacemaker market.

NUCLEAR BATTERIES

The ultimate source of terrestrial energy is the sun's nuclear activity. Humanity has succeeded in emulating it in atom bombs and in nuclear power reactors. Nature has more satisfactorily used it directly to provide our rainfall and our seasons, and has used it indirectly to generate bio-mass energy for short-term use in our wood-burning stoves and for longer term use as oil, gas, coal, and peat.

Nuclear reactions deliver up their energy in three ways. Nuclear *fission* powers both our power reactors and the "A" bomb. Nuclear *fusion* is the source of the sun's energy and powers our "H" bombs (see chapter 11). Most radioactive nuclides decay eventually to inert forms and give up energy in their decay. Nuclear *decay* seems to be the only one of these three that is suitable for small milliwatt sources.

Half-Life

The half-life of the fuel determines both the useful life of the power source and the fuel loading necessary to achieve that life. Isotopic sources degrade in an exponential fashion.

Plutonium, with a half-life of 87 years, will degrade about 16 percent in twenty-two years. Thus it needs about 20 percent extra fuel to insure full end-of-life capability after twenty years. This extra loading increases both nuclear radiation and waste heat during early years, but it is unavoidable because of the uncontrollability of the nuclear decay reaction. (Such control is achieved in fission reactors by inserting or withdrawing carbon "control" rods into or out of the fuel). With promethium, the situation is much worse. With a half-life of only two-and-a-half years, the fuel loading must be increased 400 percent to insure an adequate useful life of only ten years. This brings unwanted radiation up to unacceptable levels. With such a short half-life, this power source is not really competitive with pluto-nium. Rather, it competes with the newer, long-life chemical power sources such as lithium. The latter are less expensive, have no radiation, and therefore, no regulatory requirements. Thus, the promethium "beta cell" for pacemakers is no longer produced.

The half-life of tritium (H_3, radioactive hydrogen) is thirteen years and is probably nearer the ideal. It is also much less toxic than either plutonium or promethium. Thus, it is nearly an uncontrolled substance as far as government regulatory considerations are concerned. However, being a gas, it is prohibitively voluminous. Also, because it is very low in energy, there are formidable problems in converting its seventeen elec-trons into usable electricity. Fractional microwatt power has been successfully generated[20] by absorbing the tritium into a titanium substrate, but this is still two orders of magnitude below that needed for even the most primitive pacemaker. We carried investigations of this material through to an issued patent,[21] but the success of lithium-powered pacemakers has removed our original incentive.

PRACTICAL NUCLEAR BATTERIES

Plutonium[238] (Pu) is an alpha (helium ion) emitter. Its high velocity ions impact on the container wall and generate heat. The heat passes through the container wall and is converted into electric energy by means of thermopiles of dissimilar "P" or "N" doped bismuth telluride. The energy output of the isotope is heat. This eliminates the need of an electrical feed-through insulator through the primary fuel containment, as is required with the promethium[147] (Pm) "beta cell" design. Such a feed-through necessarily weakens the container. Since the helium pressure may build as high as 300 atmospheres during the life of the battery, container strength is a major design consideration, and Pm[147] as a pacemaker power source was abandoned long ago.

The primary disadvantage of the Pu[238] pacemaker is the toxicity of the fuel and the excessively long half-life. A microgram of the fuel in the bloodstream could be fatal. A lost nuclear pacemaker is still a hazard a millennium later. Thus, severe government regulatory control is exerted to insure that no such device is ever lost.

Early atomic pacemakers used metallic plutonium. Since this material is liable to ignite spontaneously on exposure to air, accidental exposure to air could cause a serious hazard. Thus, detailed specifications were written to insure that the enclosures could survive any "credible" accident, such as an airplane crash, being struck by a bullet, cremation, and so on. Any accident that the structure could not withstand, such as the impact of a high-velocity rifle, was arbitrarily termed "incredible." More recent nuclear pacemakers use plutonium oxide, which is a ceramic and represents far less of a hazard, should the enclosure be penetrated. However, many of the older units are still in service. With an eighty-nine-year half-life, in younger people, they may well be around for a long time.

Yet, with all its theoretical hazards, experience has shown the Pu[238] nuclear pacemaker to be the most reliable pacemaking system ever built. Such pacemakers are unquestionably safe. The patient gets less radiation than residents of Denver, where solar nuclear radiation is so poorly filtered out by the rare atmosphere that it exceeds the radiation received from a nuclear pacemaker.

THE WAY IT WAS

Dr. Alan Herman at Jet Propulsion Laboratory (JPL) did a great deal of work on exotic batteries in the early years. Their work led to a number of papers and patents. They tried a number of iodine charge transfer complexes with a number of alloys. They made one evaluation of a magnesium-lithium alloy with an iodine complex at our old Wurlitzer facility, as Herman did not have adequate dry room facilities at the lab. When the JPL cell systems were hermetically sealed at Wurlitzer, they gradually dried out and ceased to work. Evidently the properties Herman found in this preparation were due to water contamination. What was missed was the ion mobility of lithium ions from alloys of high lithium content under anhydrous (water-free/dry) conditions.

* * *

A playful employee at our old Wurlitzer facility in North Tonawanda dropped a piece of metallic lithium into a toilet during his break. The resulting violent reaction terrified him and he flushed it down the toilet, whereupon the toilet promptly blew apart with a loud noise and much smoke.

We decided to fire the employee, but he never came back from break. The local newspaper published the story with a headline "Write your own caption."

If we were still saddled with the two-year life of mercury pacemakers, all pacemakers would have gone nuclear by now. However, the advent of long-life, highly reliable lithium power sources, without regulatory problems, soon eclipsed the nuclear pacemaker and nuclear pacemakers never grew to be as much as 1 percent of the annual total used. They are no longer being made.

LITHIUM BATTERIES

The battery most used in pacemakers today is the lithium iodine cell. Also, lithium is combined with many other cathode materials by various manufacturers. It is the most active of all the alkali metals. It is rather easily handled and all the new pacemaker systems use it. The new systems differ from each other principally in their cathodes and electrolytes.

LITHIUM IODIDE BATTERIES

The first lithium battery to appear in pacemakers and by far the most used today is the lithium iodine system, invented by James Moser[22] and first introduced into pacemaker work by our group.[23] The reactions are:

$$Li \rightarrow Li^+ + e^-$$
$$I_2 + 2\ e^- \rightarrow 2\ I^-$$

The combined reaction is:

$$2\ Li + I_2 \rightarrow 2\ LiI$$

The cathode material is a complex of iodine and poly2vinylpyridine (P2VP), neither of which is a conductor of electricity. But, when mixed together and held at 300°F for three days, they react into a black viscous paste which is electronically conductive. When this paste is brought into contact with metallic lithium, a monomolecular layer of crystalline lithium iodide forms. This material is actually a molecular semiconductor which can pass lithium ions, but not iodine molecules. Since this separator forms spontaneously, it is also self-healing, tremendously increasing the reliability of the cell over the older zinc mercury cell with its vulnerable fabricated separator. It is interesting to note that pure, dry lithium iodide will not pass lithium in this form. The "molecular holes" are critical.

At the beginning-of-life the lithium iodide electrolyte impedance rises more or less linearly during the first phase of discharge and is much greater in magnitude than the cathode impedance. In the second phase of discharge, the cathode becomes starved of iodine and develops a higher impedance than the lithium iodide electrolyte. This produces the shoulder of the discharge curve, after which the loaded voltage falls more rapidly with discharge. If the load is removed for a reasonable period (three days) during phase one or phase two of discharge, the open-circuit voltage (OCV) of the cell will return to within millivolts of its original 2.8V level. During the third phase, the concentration of available iodine in the cathode has dropped so low that the Nernst equation is no longer satisfied for the 2.8v level and OCV begins to drop. This third phase is well beyond the normal design end-of-life of the cell.

The three principal zinc-mercury problems are nonexistent in the lithium iodine cell: 1) There is no gas generation. 2) There is no fabricated separator. 3) Also, because there is no gas generation, the lithium iodine cell can be hermetically sealed in a metal can with a glass-metal feed through. No body moisture can get in and no battery effluents can

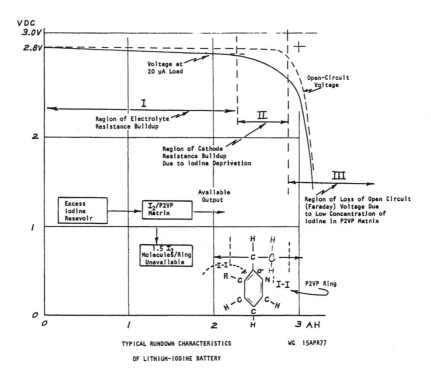

TYPICAL RUNDOWN CHARACTERISTICS   WG 15APR77

OF LITHIUM-IODINE BATTERY

Typical low-rate, triple-phase rundown pattern of lithium iodine battery.

get out. A true hermetic seal will not pass more than 30 x 10^{-9} cc of helium per second, after an overnight bomb at 60psig of helium. This is an extreme test of a good seal. No organic material will meet this test. Thus, a true hermetic seal can be achieved only with glass, metal, or ceramic materials.

We noted above that the lithium iodine cell has no fabricated separator. When lithium comes into contact with the iodine complex, a monomolecular layer of lithium iodide spontaneously forms. Should it be pierced or shattered for any reason, new lithium iodide will form to replace it. The separator is thus self-healing. These three factors permit a pacemaker cell that has a proven reliability orders of magnitude better than the older zinc-mercury battery.

Our first lithium cells (702C, 702P) used a single plate of lithium with iodine complex on one side. This proved to have too high an interface impedance, which passed beyond acceptable limits (50K ohms) before the active battery materials were exhausted. However, many of these 1972 cells were still in service after ten years. In subsequent designs this problem was solved through use of a double-sided anode structure, with iodine complex on each side of the lithium anode. The doubling of the anode surface area halved the current density. It also halved the rate of lithium iodide buildup, resulting in a cell impedance one-quarter of that of the older design.

The resistance of the cathode (phase two of rundown) is a nonlinear function of the iodine concentration in the P2VP complex. The conductance maximizes at an iodine concentration of about eight-to-one. Thus lithium batteries are built to fall to the right of the peak. As iodine is used, the operating point progresses back through the peak and then falls modestly. Thus the cathode operates at maximum conduction throughout most of its life.

Newer lithium iodine (LiI) designs strive for more and more concentrated active materials and larger anode surface areas, resulting in lower impedance. It was found at an early date[24] that multiple coatings of P2VP on the anode surface markedly reduced the interface impedance. Most LiI cells now use three coats. Corrugating or forming ridges into the anode increased anode area and decreased its impedance. In one case (the designs of Catalyst Research Corporation in 1982) two complete anode structures with four anode surfaces were used to provide another X4 reduction in impedance. All these, however, produce smaller increments of improvement as the LiI technology improves. In my opinion future requirements for milliampere pulses probably foretell liquid electrolytes and fabricated separators.

With the advent of lithium power sources, the pacemaker battery was no longer a significant problem. The heart electrode had emerged as the principal pacemaker failure mechanism. Nearly all surgical interventions today are electrode related.

ACCELERATED DISCHARGE DATA (ADD SYSTEM)

In older battery systems, such as zinc-mercury, it was common practice to discharge cells at accelerated rates and then to extrapolate the results to low rates of discharge. Such acceleration may give acceptable projections, but one must recognize that the battery chemistry may follow different paths at different rates and that internal self-discharge may well be masked by rapid rundown. In the case of zinc-mercury, rapid rundown in weeks gave capacities comparable to rundown at six-month rates, but missed the internal self-discharge at 37°C that limited the life of such cells to an average life of two years.

Early observations suggested that data from accelerating the rundown of lithium iodine cells was of minimal value. The impedance of early cells was so high that it soon exceeded the value of the test load resistor and became in itself current-limiting. Later cells had double anodes and lower impedance, and John Greenwood[25] was able to show a close correlation between accelerated discharge data and that obtained in real-time rundown at low rates. His method consisted of dividing a group of about fifty randomly selected batteries into six or seven groups. Each group was discharged at a different rate (load resistors of 4K to 133K ohms). When the first group became discharged, its performance was extrapolated linearly to a projected discharge curve at a nominal 140K ohm load (20 uA at 2.8V). As each subsequent group became discharged, it, too, was projected and superimposed on the previous data. Thus, each successive group added a correction to the predictive curve. This produced a very early estimate of the cells predicted performance with the accuracy of the prediction improving with each correction. The equation to project the actual data to the 140K ohms load curve is derived in the chapter 4 appendix, at the end of this volume.

In addition, another lot of fifty cells was put on test at a load of 100K ohms to provide a larger sample at a rate nearer to the specified rate. We have included a sample evaluation of one battery design to show the operation of the ADD system.

We selected a high-production cell design for an example of the ADD process. The WGLtd. Model 761/23 design was probably the most used pacemaker battery in 1985. In 1980–1983, over 140,000 cells were provided to twelve pacemaker manufacturers in six different countries for use in many different pacemaker models.

In 1978, either five or six cells each were put on loads of 4.53K, 6.98K, 16.5K, 37.5K, 73.2K and 133K. Fifty cells were put on a load of 100K ohms. Thus, more than ninety cells were tested. At 1,632 days, all of the cells on loads up to 16.5K were exhausted, as was one cell on 35.7K load (33 cells total). All the other cells were still on test.

Table 1 shows minimum-mean-maximum values of MAHR, V_R and the mean of V_{140K} predictions for each load value. The rated capacity of this cell is 2.5 AH.

Table 2 shows the combined mean predicted values of V_{140K} for all load values at eight points on the discharge curve, and the days on test needed to arrive at each point.

In evaluating Table 2, means, heavy-load data, near end-of-life of the cell (that above and to the right of the dashed line) have been deleted as more moderate-load data became available.* The heavy-load data are a somewhat poorer approximation near end-of-life. The inclu-

TABLE 1
MEASURED MAHR, V_R, AND CALCULATED V_{140K}

MAHR		800	1200	1600	2000	2200	2300	2400	2450	2500
R=4.53K										
	min	780	1164	1536	1943	2134	2134	--	--	--
MAHR	mean	808	1198	1594	2017	2159	2159	--	--	--
	max	819	1225	1676	2045	2278	2278	--	--	--
	min	2372	1847	1061	581	323		186	--	--
V_R	mean	2432	2009	1163	588	381		263	--	--
	max	2525	2072	1259	602	437		334	--	--
V_{140K} mean		2786	2764	2677	2496	2330		2114	--	--
R = 6.98K										
	min	791	1117	1552	1930	2105		2328	--	--
MAHR	mean	799	1196	1598	2014	2208		2413	--	--
	max	804	1211	1634	2077	2266		2458	--	--
	min	2544	2325	1719	926	699		249	--	--
V_R	mean	2600	2450	1890	1005	737		332	--	--
	max	2645	2626	2040	1036	770		395	--	--
V_{140K} mean		2789	2780	2733	2570	2456		2034	--	--
R = 12.4K										
	min	805	1196	1577	1962	2152		2378	--	--
MAHR	mean	808	1200	1500	1997	2192		2405	--	--
	max	811	1200	1617	2059	2263		2460	--	--
	min	2636	2510	2045	1336	1034		427	--	--
V_R	mean	2652	2535	2180	1394	1057		600	--	--
	max	2677	2590	2363	1482	1083		734	--	--
V_{140K} mean		2786	2774	2730	2569	2443		2095	--	--
R = 16.5K										
	min	807	1207	1561	1927	2088		2298	2353	--
MAHR	mean	811	1213	1588	2002	2178		2398	2450	--
	max	816	1227	1620	2958	2242		2471	2521	--
	min	2661	2511	2061	1438	1205		739	519	--
V_R	mean	2686	2572	2290	1605	1305		824	646	--
	max	2727	2650	2440	1726	1383		898	761	--
V_{140K} mean		2786	2770	2727	2572	2466		2191	2001	--

TABLE 2
PREDICTED VALUES OF V_{140K} AT VARIOUS DISCHARGE LEVELS

"Heavy-load" data (discarded when lighter-load data became available) →

R	MAHR	800	1200	1600	2000	2200	2300	2400	2450	2500
4.53K	mv	2786	2764	2677	2496	2330	2114	--	--	--
	da	58	90	139	238	308	365	--	--	--
6.98K	mv	2789	2780	2733	2570	2456	--	2034	--	--
	da	86	132	185	273	336	--	455	--	--
12.4K	mv	2786	2774	2730	2569	2443	--	2095	--	--
	da	153	231	315	434	518	--	651	--	--
16.5K	mv	2786	2770	2727	2572	2466	--	2181	2001	--
	da	162	308	413	560	644	--	784	833	--
35.7K	mv	2783	2770	2739	2621	2487	--	2255	2168	2075
	da	427	651	875	1113	1260	--	1443	1506	1555
73.2K	mv	2782	2769	--	--	--	--	--	--	--
	da	882	1323	--	--	--	--	--	--	--
100K	mv	2784	--	--	--	--	--	--	--	--
(50 cells)	da	1127	--	--	--	--	--	--	--	--
133K	mv	2774	--	--	--	--	--	--	--	--
	da	1015	--	--	--	--	--	--	--	--
min	mv	2774	2764	2677	2496	2443	--	2095	2001	--
max	mv	2789	2780	2739	2572	2487	--	2255	2168	--
mean	mv	2784	2771	2721	2566	2436	--	2136	2085	2075
Std.Dev.	mv	±4	±5	±22	±40	±70	--	±60	±84	--

(left axis label: 365 day data)

From WGLtd. internal papers.

TABLE 3
DELIVERED CAPACITY AT EXHAUSTION

R	S/N	MAHR AT EXHAUSTION	DAYS
4.53K	10103	2405	491
	10112	2375	427
	10226	2327	426
	10240	2372	386
	10249	2403	491
	mean	2384 MAHR @ R = 4.53K	
12.4K	9828	2513	778
	10276	2494	742
	10280	2470	665
	10283	2440	679
	10292	2519	777
	10317	2499	763
	mean	2489 MAHR @ R = 12.4K	
16.5K	10385	2436	926
	10401	2510	848
	10404	2527	924
	10474	2497	875
	10476	2499	924
	10493	2563	882
	mean	2505 MAHR @ R = 16.5K	
35.7K	10512	1534	1583
	10582	*	*
	10638	*	*
	10653	*	*
	10669	*	*
	10688		
	mean	2534 MAHR @ R = 35.7K	

73.2K, 100K, 133K*

*Still on test at 1632 days, as of July 1, 1983.

Curve 1.

MODEL 761/23

CONSTANT LOAD DISCHARGE (AVERAGE CURVES)

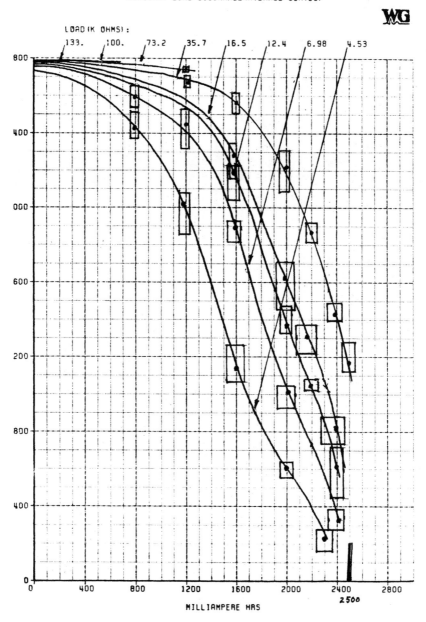

MILLIAMPERE HRS

Curve 2.   MODEL 761/23 ADD - 140K PROJECTIONS
FROM ALL LOADS: ——
FROM 100K DATA ONLY: ---

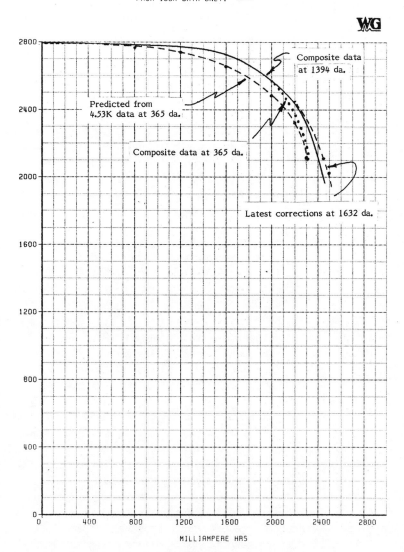

THE WAY IT WAS

MANNY VILLAFANA, Entrepreneur Extraordinaire

Manuel Villafana was born of Puerto Rican parents, was raised in the Bronx, and had the short life expectancy of a member of a Bronx youth gang. The Boys' Club rescued him and motivated him toward a useful life. Manny never forgot and is still a major supporter of the Boys' Club and of St. Jude, the patron saint of those in trouble.

My acquaintance with Manny goes back over four decades to the time during which he was employed by Picker International, selling Medtronic pacemakers to the international market. He was an aggressive, successful salesman.

When difficulties arose between Picker and Medtronic, Manny moved over to Medtronic. Not satisfied with a Minneapolis desk, he took it upon himself to build a very successful Medtronic outlet in Argentina. His fluent Spanish and his natural charm intoxicated the Argentine market. He left only when a recurring fungal infection of endemic nature threatened the life of his son.

Later, after a stint as president of Med General, making operating room lights, he returned to his first love: pacemakers. In 1970 we in Buffalo had completed our work at Medtronic and had moved on to the next great problem, pacemaker batteries. We chose the lithium iodine system and had it well into development in 1970–71. One winter day in 1970, I got a phone call from Manny. He asked if I had a passport. I said that I did. He said, "Good, meet me at JFK Friday night. We're going to Paris!" I said I couldn't because I had a paper to deliver the following Tuesday. He said, "You'll be back in time. I'll pay your way." I said, "That's different." So we went to France to sell a package to a French company. Manny worked with the sales people in Spanish while I talked for two hours, without preparation, about our batteries, in French! That was the way Manny operated.

Eventually, the package didn't work out and Manny relocated to Minneapolis to work for Cardiac Pacemakers Inc (CPI). I warned Manny that lithium was too new to risk his company on. I told him to work in mercury and then move into lithium. He said, "No. If I'm going to buck the big boys, it's got to be with something completely new, that solves all the problems, but is too risky for them to undertake." CPI implanted the first lithium pacemaker in November 1972 and overnight became a major factor in the marketplace. Manny had gambled and won.

We sold him batteries and didn't bill him for over a year. Some say that was what got CPI off to a successful financial start. We lectured at

(continued)

his sales schools and did statistical analysis on his reliability (and ours!). We backed him with papers in Japan and sent our people in to help him with interface problems. In return he gave us our first big medical exposure that proved lithium was the way to go.

One thing about Manny. Wherever he is, there's excitement and things jump. There's no way to stay in your comfortable rut when he's around. Good luck, Manny.

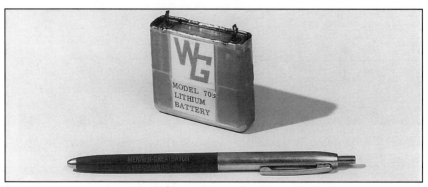

Original Model 702 Prototype Battery. (Note the rough, irregular weld, ineptly made by the author.)

sion of such data unnecessarily distorts the more moderate-load data. Thus data above the dashed line are not included in the means calculated for 2200, 2400, 2450, and 2500 MAHR at 1,632 days.

Curve 1 shows the mean data for each load group. The box around each data point includes *all* data points from that set.

Curve 2 shows the mean V_{140K} predictions from the composites on Curve 1. The first approximation at 365 days is shown, along with the corrected curve for 1,394 days, and finally, minor corrections near end-of-life, contributed by newer data, primarily from the 37.5K test, up to 1,632 days.

Several facts may be noted from the accompanying tables and curves:

1. Cells under heavy load deliver 90 percent to 95 percent of the capacity obtainable under light loads.
2. The general shape of the discharge curve is apparent from the 4.53K data within nine months. In another three months, the

*Note that this deletion is solely applicable to the example in this article and is not necessarily representative of methods used in the periodic WGLtd. "ADD" reports. Data for tables 1 and 2 comes from WGLtd. internal papers.

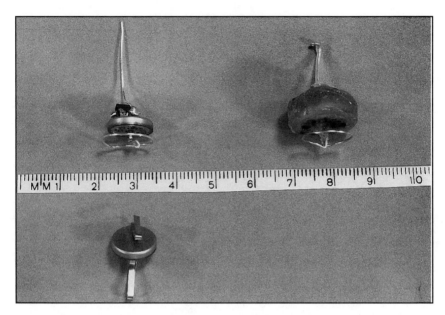

Lithium Silver Vanadium Pentoxide Button Cell, built into an infection control module for control of bacterial infection in plant clones. This model was autoclaved fifty times.

complete curve is predicted, with support corrections for the early part of the curve, from the 6.98K, 12.4K, and 16.5K data. Thus, within one year, one can conservatively predict the ten-year performance of the design.

3. Real-life performance at pacemaker loads will slightly exceed ADD predictions. To date, this excess appears to more than compensate for any internal self-discharge that may be encountered in the long-term situation.

THE LITHIUM SILVER CHROMATE CELL

There has been some use, particularly in Europe, of a pacemaker battery, built by SAFT of Potier, France. This cell uses a cathode of silver chromate, a polypropylene separator, and has an OCV of 3.35v. The liquid electrolyte is a lithium perchlorate solution in an organic solvent. The reaction is:

$$2Li + Ag_2CrO_4 \rightarrow Li_2CrO_4 + 2Ag$$

Two cells are usually used in parallel to achieve the desired capacity. This cell is not currently used in U.S. production pacemakers.

THE LITHIUM COPPER SULFIDE CELL

About four decades ago the SAFT company developed a lithium-copper sulfide cell. Cordis Corp. presently manufactures this battery under license in an in-house facility in Miami. The OCV is about 2v, and three cells are usually used in series. This cell, too, requires a fabricated separator. The reactions are:

anode: $Li \rightarrow Li^+ + e^-$

the cathode discharges in two steps:

$2CuS + 2e^- \rightarrow Cu^+ + S^=$

$Cu_2S + 2e^- \rightarrow 2Cu + S^=$

The second reaction creates a lower plateau voltage at 1.75v during the last portion of life providing an end-of-life warning indicator.

The overall cell reactions are:

$2CuS + 2Li \rightarrow Cu_2S + Li_2S$ V=2.12v

$Cu_2S + 2Li \rightarrow 2Cu + Li_2S$ V=1.75v

THE LITHIUM BROMINE/CHLORINE CELL

This cell uses a bromine-thionyl chloride complex[26] which actually has a higher OCV than either bromine or chlorine. Thus it is a new cathode, dissimilar from either. The cathode structure contains a carbon substrate. The electrolyte is lithium tetrachloraluminate. The container is a sealed stainless steel structure. The current collectors are expanded nickel screen. A "D" size cell can support a current of one ampere for over five hours. Such cells were originally built for use in military/commercial applications, but are now being designed into implantable prosthetics, such as drug delivery devices. Both this cell and the lithium sulfuryl chloride cell described below, provide energy density in excess of 1.0 watt-hour per cm^3.

THE LITHIUM SULFURYL CHLORIDE CELL

This cell is somewhat similar to the lithium bromine chlorine cell described above except for the use of sulfuryl chloride ($SO_2 Cl_2$) in place of thionyl chloride ($SOCl_2$) in the cathode.[27] The additive in this case is dissolved chlorine rather than the bromine chlorine complex. Both systems insure that no elemental sulphur will result from the battery reactions at any stage. Sulphur reacts explosively with lithium and its presence in the battery could prove hazardous if such a step were allowed to occur. The outstanding feature of the $LiSO_2Cl_2$ battery is its ability to operate safely at 150°C temperature. One commercial use for it is in instrumentation at the bottom of oil well drill holes. Such a property insures that it can be safely autoclaved.

THE LITHIUM SILVER VANADIUM OXIDE (SVO™) CELL

The anode is lithium and the cathode is silver vanadium oxide[28] or, more properly, AgV_xO_y. The electrolyte is lithium perchlorate in a propylene carbonate solvent. We have used this cell in small structures to fit in a test tube. The cell powered a constant-current generator which delivered one microampere to corrode a silver anode to provide a bacteriocidal environment for infected plant clones. We recently autoclaved several such devices fifty times without battery damage.

We have also used a larger version (2.0 AH) to power an autoclavable, fixed-rate pacemaker pulse generator of unique design. We had autoclaved this device eleven times by 1983. We believe that this cell design will prove useful in many prosthetic implants where autoclavability is desirable.

The SVO cell offers five features that demonstrate its attractiveness for implant work.

1) The beginning-of-life voltage is 3.2v which gradually falls to an end-of-life voltage of 2.0v. This is somewhat higher than that of LiI.
2) It is capable of ampere pulses. This is the battery of choice for implantable cardioverters/defibrillators and its principle use in 2000 is in this service.
3) The cell can be made repeatably autoclavable. We have autoclaved button cells of this chemistry fifty times without change in characteristics.

4) The open-circuit-voltage (OCV) is dependent on remaining life. It has a rundown which is characterized by a well-defined fall in OCV during discharge. This permits a rather reliable indication of remaining battery life by means of simply measuring either the battery voltage.

5) The chemistry is a very forgiving one, reminiscent of the familiar LiI reliability. The cell is short-circuit proof. It will neither vent nor rupture under short-circuit conditions up to temperatures of 50°C.

LITHIUM CARBON MONOFLOURIDE CELL

The LiCFX cell is seeing use in some commercial applications. There are some indications that it may be autoclavable, if properly packaged. Also, its OCV of 3.2v is very attractive. Like the SVO™ and LiI cells, it is a comparatively safe chemistry. We must *always* remember, however, that all cathodes are strong reducers and anytime lithium melts in a battery, an accident may result. Some lithium battery chemistries have an energy content equal to dynamite. It is an understatement to say that eternal vigilance is the price of the safe manufacture and operation of lithium battery systems. The LiCFX system appears to be a worthy successor to the venerable LiI system in pacemakers that require more current capacity due to extended functions like telemetry, extended memory, and some therapeutic functions.

CONCLUSION

We have presented a historical and technical review of pacemaker power sources as they have been used in pacemakers over the past forty years. We have tried to demonstrate their strong points and their weak points and to show how the historical development was related to the techno-logical need. It is interesting to note that, after the first zinc-mercury battery, most of the designs originated in the medical field rather than in the commercial, military, or aerospace field. The performance and reliability requirements of medical implantable prosthetic devices often transcend those of the traditional high-reliability fields. The human body is a very hostile environment, far more so than space or the bottom of the sea.

We have tried also to show how the technological development of pacemakers and other prosthetic devices required a similar develop-mental effort in battery design. At times, battery design lagged behind and the battery became the limiting factor in the performance or the reliability of the device. Fortunately, over the last decade, the battery seems to have stayed ahead, and the limitation on pacemaker performance and reliability today, although still chemical to a degree, is not the battery. Another fascinating field of body electrochemistry is the physiological polarization of implanted electrodes. This, along with the electrode structure itself, has brought the cardiac electrode to the forefront as the limiting factor in pacemaker performance and reliability.

NOTES

1. J. Moser, "Solid State Lithium-iodine Battery." U.S. Patent #3,660,163, 1970.

2. Ibid.

3. W. Greatbatch, J. Lee, W. Mathias, M. Eldridge, J. Moser, and A. Schneider, "The Solid State Lithium Battery." *IEEE BME Transactions* 18, no. 5 (1971): 317.

4. W. Greatbatch and T. Bustard, "A PuO Nuclear Power Source for Implantable Cardiac Pacemakers." *IEEE Trans. BME* 20, no. 5 (1973): 332.

5. W. Greatbatch, R. Mead, R. McLean, F. Rudolph, and W. Frenz, "Lithium Bromine Cell." U.S. Patent 3,994,747, 1976.

6. R. Murphy, P. Krehl, and C. Liang, "The Effect of Halogen Addition on the Performance Characteristics of Lithium/Sulfur Oxychloride Battery Systems." *Proc 16th Intersoc. Energy Engin. Conf.* (ASME) 1 (1980): 97.

7. C. Liang et al., "Metal Oxide Composite Cathode Material for High Energy Density Batteries." U.S. Patent 4,310,609, 1982.

8. Ibid.

9. S. Ruben, "Balanced Alkaline Dry Cells," *Trans. Electrochem. Soc.* 92 (1947): 183.

10. Ibid.

11. W. M. Chardack et al., "Experience with an Implantable Pacemaker." *Ann. N.Y. Acad. Sci.* 111 (1964): 1075–92.

12. S. Furman and D. Escher, "Transtelephone Pacemaker Monitoring." *Ann. Thoracic Surg.* 20, no. 3 (1975): 22; S. Furman, "Cardiac Pacing: An Endless Frontier." *Medical Instrumentation* (AAMI) 7, no. 3 (1973): 168.

13. W. Greatbatch and W. Chardack, "A Transistorized Implantable Pacemaker for the Long-term Correction of Complete Heart Block." *Trans. NEREM Conf.,* Boston 1 (1959): 8; W. Chardack, A. Gage, and W. Greatbatch, "A Transistorized, Self-contained, Implantable Pacemaker for the Long-term Correction of Complete Heart Block." *Surgery* 48, no. 4 (1960): 643.

14. P. Racine and H. Massie, "An Experimental Internally Powered Cardiac Pacemaker." *Med. Res. Engin.* 5, no. 3 (1966).

15. O. Roy, J. Armour, W. Firor, R. Wehnert, D. Macgregor, K. Sindhavenada, and W. Bigelow, "A Batteryless Biological Cardiovascular Pacemaker." *Am. College of Surgery Forum* 17 (1966): 164.

16. M. Schaldach, "Implantable Electrochemical Energy Sources." *Proc. 9th Intl. Conf. MBE,* Melbourne 8 (1971).

17. J. Cywinski, Personal communication, 1980.

18. S. Furman et al., "Transtelephone Pacemaker Monitoring."

19. A. Senning, "Problems in the Use of Pacemakers." *J. Cardiovasc. Surg.* 5 (1964): 651.

20. F. Gatt, "A Tritium Pacemaker Battery Design." *Proc. 9th Intl. Conf.* MBE, Melbourne, 1971.

21. W. Greatbatch, "Device for Converting Nuclear Energy into Electrical Energy." U.S. Patent 3,836,798, 1974.

22. J. Moser, "Solid State Lithium-iodine Battery."

23. W. Greatbatch et al., "A PuO Nuclear Power Source for Implantable Cardiac Pacemakers."

24. R. Mead, "The Effect of Multiple coats of P2VP on Lithium Anode Impedance." WGLtd. internal memo, 1976.

25. J. Greenwood, "Accelerated Discharge Data (ADD)." WGLtd. internal paper, 1980.

26. R. Murphy, P. Krehl, and C. Liang, "The Effect of Halogen Addition on the Performance Characteristics of Lithium/Sulfur Oxychloride Battery Systems." *Proc 16th Intersoc. Energy Engin. Conf.* (ASME) 1 (1980): 97.

27. C. Liang, "Metal Oxide Composite Cathode Material for High Energy Density Batteries."

28. Ibid.

5

STATISTICAL EVALUATION OF DEVICE RELIABILITY

STATISTICAL EVALUATION OF BATTERY LONGEVITY

The failure rate for most devices may be classified into three distinct categories. During early life, some failures occur during burn-in. A long service period then follows during which failures are linearly and randomly scattered. Lastly, towards end-of-life (EOL), a period follows where failure rate increases greatly due to exhaustion or wearout. A graph of such performance characteristics resembles a bathtub and is labeled as such by reliability engineers. In pacemaker pulse generators and in implantable batteries, the burn-in period will be a few weeks while the service life may be five to eight years. The EOL period will vary greatly from battery to battery depending on battery size, the power requirements of ancillary functions such as programming or telemetry interrogation, and on the number of times the pacemaker was inhibited by the "demand" function and thus not required to deliver its usual energy pulse to the heart. However, a typical EOL period might be one or two years.

The improving reliability and longevity of pacemakers have produced a growing need for a standardized method of evaluation of pacemaker pulse generators and their power supplies. We have adapted two standard statistical techniques to attain this objective: 1) cumulative survival analysis (sometimes referred to as the "actuarial" method) gives an unconditional standardized measure of past performance; and 2) random linear failure analysis, which will predict future performance from past exposure, even if no failures have yet occurred, but it requires

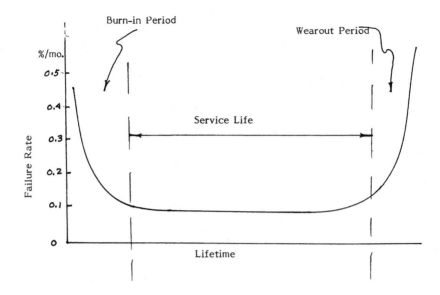

Bathtub curve, measuring the lifespan of a pacemaker, including the time when it is usable for the patient.

an assumption that failures, when and if they do occur, will be randomly and linearly scattered. It is applicable only during the service life and not during burn-in or during wearout.

CUMULATIVE SURVIVAL ANALYSIS

Berkson et al. made the first medical use of cumulative survival analysis at the Mayo Clinic to evaluate the survival of cancer patients.[1] This technique, however, has long been used in the insurance field and is known there as the actuarial method. A. Schaudig et al. used it in Munich for pacemaker evaluation,[2] and G. Green independently and intuitively developed some elements of this system.[3] In this chapter, we will use much of Schaudig's methodology, but with Green's terminology.

The usefulness of cumulative survival analysis lies in the fact that it evaluates only the performance of exposed units. It does this in such a way that the results are relatively independent of any bias on the part of the data taker. It is important, however, to precisely define each status class. Failure status in particular must be carefully defined. Our own definition interprets it from the patient's point of view as a malfunction, after wound closure, that requires additional surgical intervention.

Others may disagree with our definition, and perhaps rightly so. However, a pulse generator whose output has dropped 50 percent but still paces is functional from the patient's point of view. A malfunction that requires surgical intervention, however, is quite another matter. We will show here that three pacemaker series, from three different countries and three different doctors, using two different pacemakers, all showed the same cumulative survival, i.e., twelve to fifteen months at 90 percent cumulative survival. The reason is that they all used the same battery, which was the principal cause of failure.

In cumulative survival analysis, individual quarterly failure rates and quarterly survival rates are calculated for exposed units only. The quarterly survival rates are then successively multiplied by each other, forming a cumulative survival. The output of the analysis is the number of months at which a specified percentage of the exposed units survive. We calculate this for 90 percent and 50 percent cumulative survival. Experience has shown that the quarterly failure rate breaks sharply upward somewhere between these two limits and the point of the break is perhaps a good "elective replacement time" (ERT).

We use Green's terminology for identifying status.

A) *Incomplete lifetime*: units that have attained the particular age indicated and are still implanted and operating satisfactorily. The value of A indicates the maturity of the series. If all A = 0, then the series is completely matured, i.e., out of service.

B) *Curtailed lifetime*: units removed at the indicated age for reasons unrelated to unit malfunction. Such reasons might be unrelated death, electrode problem, pulse generator erosion, and so on.

C) *Elective lifetime*: no system fault. We generally class these with B, curtailed lifetime.

D) *Failed lifetime*: a unit removed sometime after wound closure because of unit malfunction. Note that we reserve the word "failure" for a clinical failure. We prefer the word "malfunction" to describe a unit that has specification. We feel that the decision as to whether a "malfunction" is sufficiently severe to justify removal as a "failure" is a medical one that the physician should remain free to make.

As an example, let us examine data for Green's series of older mercury-powered pacemaker pulse generators from 1968–1970 (Table 1). Data are divided horizontally into quarterly periods and vertically into ten columns. M is the number of months. N is the total number of units that entered the quarter (i.e.; became that old). Obviously any unit used entered the first quarter so that N1 is the total number of units in the

TABLE 1

CUMULATIVE SURVIVAL OF 162 MEDTRONIC 5870/5841 MERCURY PACEMAKERS, 1968–1970

(M) Age (Months)	(N) Number of units	(A) Incomplete lifetime	(B) Curtailed lifetime	(D) Failed units	(T) Total A+B+D	(X) Exposed units X=N–T/2	(F) Fraction failed F=D/X	(S) Fraction survived S=1–F	(S1) Cumulative survival S1=S1×S
0-3	162	8	14	0	22	151	0	1.000	1.000
3-6	140	13	9	0	22	129	0	1.000	1.000
6-9	118	9	4	1	14	111.5	0.009	0.992	0.992
9-12	104	5	2	2	9	101.5	0.020	0.980	0.971
12-15	95	9	3	3	15	89	0.034	0.966	0.938
15-18	80	7	2	5	14	75.7	0.067	0.934	0.874
18-21	66	5	2	4	11	58.5	0.068	0.931	0.815
21-24	55	11	0	4	15	49.5	0.081	0.919	0.749
24-27	40	14	1	6	21	32.5	0.184	0.815	0.610
27-30	19	5	1	7	13	16	0.438	0.563	0.343
30-33	6	1	0	2	3	4	0.500	0.500	0.172
33-36	3	1	0	1	2	3	0.333	0.667	0.114
36-39	1	0	0	1	1	0.5			
39-42	0								
42-45									
45-48									
48-51									
51-54									
54-57									
57-60									
Total		88	38	36	162	(807.5) × 3 = 2422.5 Pacemaker months			

Adapted from Green, "Progress in Pacemaker Technology." *J. Electrocardiol.* 7, no. 4 (1974).

series (162 in this case). *A* is the number of units that have attained the age indicated and are still working satisfactorily. Thus A1 = 8, indicating that 8 units are between zero and three months old and still working at the time of this evaluation. *B* is the number of units removed for reasons unrelated to pulse generator malfunction. B1 = 14, so 14 unfailed units were removed in their first three months of life. Thus a total of 22 units did not see a full three months service. Therefore only 140 units (N2) entered the second quarter. Thus, N2 = N1 - T1. Because the 22 units were not exposed a full three months, we average them and say that the exposed units (X) were 162 - 22/2 = 151 units. Thus X I = N I - (A+B)/2.

The first failure occurred in the third quarter. In this quarter 111.5 units were exposed so that the quarterly failure rate was F3 = 0.009, or 0.9 percent per quarter. Quarterly survival rate is S = (1 - F), or 0.992. The next quarter, two more units failed, giving a quarterly survival rate of 0.980. This, multiplied by the previous cumulative survival rate of 0.992, gives a cumulative survival of 0.971. Thus the table grows until N goes to zero. In practice, the cumulative survival becomes of questionable significance when X drops under 30 units. At this point digitization error will produce a 3 percent drop in cumulative survival for a single additional failure. Column A will move downward with age and will dissipate to the right into B or D. Existing entries in B and D however will stay there, increasing if A is not zero, but not decreasing.

Tables 2 and 3 show the cumulative survival analysis on two additional series from Schaudig in Munich[4] and from Furman in New York.[5] These two series are contemporary with that of Green in Table 1. The three series add up to a total of 490 pacemaker pulse generators. The three series, compared to each other, show a 90 percent cumulative survival of fifteen months plus or minus one quarter, and a 50 percent cumulative survival at thirty to thirty-three months plus or minus one quarter. This is an impressive consistency from such geographically disparate data sets. The reason of course is that the same battery, the Mallory RM1 cell, was the principal failure mode in all three series.

Indications of Departure from Randomness

Green's series is only half mature, with 88 A-type units still at risk out of a total of 162. Nevertheless, examination of column F is interesting. Up until twenty-four months, the quarterly failure rate ranged from 0 to 8 percent per quarter, but in the ninth quarter it jumped to 18 percent and continued to increase. This sharp break upward could be regarded as a signal of the desirability of imminent elective replacement. We seem to see such a signal in most series and it always falls somewhere between 90 percent and 50 percent cumulative survival.

TABLE 2.

CUMULATIVE SURVIVAL OF 227 CORDIS ECTICOR MERCURY PACEMAKERS, 1969–1971

(M) Age (Months)	(N) Number of units	(A) Incomplete lifetime	(B) Curtailed lifetime	(D) Failed units	(T) Total units A+B+D	(X) Exposed units X=N−T/2	(F) Fraction failed F=D/X	(S) Fraction survived S=1−F	(S1) Cumulative survival S1=S1×S
0-3	227	0	17	4	21	218.5	0.018	0.982	0.982
3-6	204	0	10	1	11	199	0.005	0.995	0.977
6-9	193	0	7	2	9	189.5	0.011	0.989	0.966
9-12	184	0	12	4	16	178	0.023	0.977	0.944
12-15	168	0	9	4	13	163.5	0.025	0.975	0.921
15-18	155	0	8	9	17	150	0.061	0.939	0.864[a]
18-21	138	0	13	7	20	131.5	0.055	0.945	0.817
21-24	118	0	15	19	34	108.5	0.175	0.825	0.674
24-27	84	0	18	10	28	75	0.133	0.867	0.584
27-30	56	0	11	12	23	50.5	0.237	0.762	0.445[b]
30-33	33	0	8	10	18	29	0.345	0.655	0.292
33-36	15	0	2	3	5	14	0.357	0.643	0.188
36-39	10	0	1	0	1	9.5	0	1.000	0.188
39-42	9	0	2	1	3	8.0	0.133	0.867	0.169
42-45	6	0	1	2	3	5.5	0.444	0.555	0.094
45-48	3	0	0	0	0	3	0		
48-51	3	0	0	0	0	3	0	1.000	0.094
51-54	3	0	2	0	2	2	0	1.000	0.094
54-57	1	0	1	0	1	0.5	0	1.000	0.094
57-60	0								
Total		0	137	88	225	1497.5 × 3 = 4492.5 Pacemaker months			

Adapted from Schaudig and Zimmerman, "Comparison of Function Time of Different Pacemaker Systems." *Ann. Cardiol.* 20, no. 4 (1971).

a. 90 percent cumulative survival.

b. 50 percent cumulative survival.

TABLE 3
CUMULATIVE SURVIVAL OF 101 CORDIS 143E MERCURY PACEMAKERS, 1970–1973

(M) Age (Months)	(N) Number of units	(A) Incomplete lifetime	(B) Curtailed lifetime	(D) Failed units	(T) Total units A+B+D	(X) Exposed units X=N−T/2	(F) Fraction failed F=D/X	(S) Fraction survived S=1−F	(S1) Cumulative survival S1=S1×S
0-3	101	0	9	0	9	96.5	0.000	1.000	1.000
3-6	92	0	0	0	0	92.0	0.000	1.000	1.000
6-9	92	0	9	2	11	87.5	0.023	0.977	0.977
9-12	81	0	2	3	5	80.0	0.037	0.962	0.940
12-15	76	0	3	4	7	74.5	0.054	0.946	0.890[a]
15-18	69	2	1	2	5	67.5	0.030	0.970	0.864
18-21	64	1	1	0	2	63.0	0.000	1.000	0.864
21-24	62	1	0	2	3	61.5	0.033	0.967	0.836
24-27	59	2	3	9	14	56.5	0.159	0.841	0.702
27-30	45	2	0	5	7	44.0	0.114	0.886	0.623
30-33	38	2	3	4	9	35.5	0.113	0.887	0.552
33-36	29	5	0	4	9	26.5	0.151	0.849	0.469[b]
36-39	20	8	0	2	10	16.0	0.125	0.875	0.410
39-42	10	6	0	0	6	7.0	0.000	1.000	0.410
42-45	4	1	2	1	4	2.5	0.400	0.600	0.246
Totals		30	33	38	101	(810.5)3 = 2431.5 Pacemaker			

months/N = 24.1 months average

Adapted from Furman et al., "Implantable Cardiac Pacemakers: Status Report and Resource Guideline (ICHD)." *Circulation* 50 (1974).

[a] 90% Cumulative survival at beginning of quarter.
[b] 50% Cumulative survival at beginning of quarter.

Table 4 represents a more modern series of 795 lithium-powered CPI pacemakers from which the author had the privilege of personally analyzing the raw data. Cumulative survival analysis for Table 4 is unrewarding because of the immaturity of the series, both because of the short time the units have been implanted and because of the obvious superiority of the lithium batteries in this series over the zinc-mercury batteries in Green's series. To analyze the lithium data, we have chosen a second method: random linear failure analysis.

RANDOM LINEAR FAILURE ANALYSIS

Table 4 shows a pattern typical of newer pacemaker series. If early mortality (failures at one week or less) are ignored, the failure pattern looks relatively random. If such an assumption is valid, a new branch of mathematical analysis is open to us. D. Rosenbaum et al. used the

TABLE 4

CUMULATIVE SURVIVAL OF 795 LITHIUM IODINE PACEMAKERS, 1972–1974

(M) Age (Months)	(N) Number of units	(A) Incomplete lifetime	(B) Curtailed lifetime	(D) Failed units	(T) Total A+B+D	(X) Exposed units X=N−T/2	(F) Fraction failed F=D/X	(S) Fraction survived S=1−F	(S1) Cumulative survival S1=S1×S
0-3	795	3	17	5	25	786.0	0.006	0.994	0.994
3-6	770	22	10	1	33	754.0	0.001	0.999	0.992
6-9	737	165	6	0	171	651.5	0	1.000	0.992
9-12	566	240	0	1	241	446.0	0.002	0.998	0.990
12-15	325	198	2	0	200	225.0	0	1.000	0.990
15-18	125	74	0	0	74	88.0	0	1.000	0.990
18-21	51	32	0	1	33	35.0	0.02	0.971	0.961
21-24	18	16	0	0	16	10.0	0	1.000	0.961
24-27	2	2	0	0	2	1.0	0	1.000	0.961
27-30									
Totals		752	35	8	795				

TABLE 5
CONFIDENCE LEVEL IN A 0.1% PER MONTH FAILURE RATE
FOR 795 PC. LITHIUM-IODINE PACEMAKERS, CLINICALLY IMPLANTED.

$$C = 1 - \sum_{r=0}^{r=R} F_r$$

Where: $F_r = \dfrac{(PN)^r}{r!}(1-P)^{N-r}$

And: P = Desired failure rate   = .001
          N = Pacemaker months of exposure   = 8990
          R = Number of random failures   = 5

Type Value of R: (Number of Failures)
? 5
Type Value of N: (Number of Pacemaker Months Exposure)
? 8990
Desired Monthly Failure Rate ?
? .001

Coefficients F0 to F9 for Individual Quarterly Failure Rates are:
1.24086E-4   1.11665 E-3   5.02438E-3   1 .50715E-2   3.3907 E-2   6.10258E-2
0   0   0   0
The confidence level in a 0.1% per month failure rate is 88.37%.

---

technique of random linear failure analysis to arrive at a longevity design target for nuclear-powered pacemakers.[6] This method is particularly useful in situations where few or no failures exist and no failure pattern is discernible.

The confidence level (C) in a given maximum failure rate (P) for (R) failures in (N) pacemaker months of exposure can be derived as:

$$C = 1 - \sum \frac{(PN)^r}{r!}(1-P)^{N-r}$$

summed iteratively over all the values of r from 0 to R. Rosenbaum suggested a P value of 0.15 percent per month; for example, six failures out of 100 pacemakers in 40 months, or 94 percent survival. Since that time both lithium and nuclear pacemaker systems have demonstrated far better reliability that this, but let us assume a design target of 0.1 percent per month failure rate and examine the 795 lithium pacemakers in Table 2. Of the first five units which failed in the first quarter, three failed in the first week and are eliminated from the calculation. Thus the total number of failures to be counted are 5 rather than the 8 shown in the table. Thus, R = 5, N = 3, X = 8990, and P = 0.001. Then:

$$C = 1 - \sum \frac{(0.001[8990])^r}{r!} (0.999)^{8990-r} = 88\%$$

Table 5 shows a computer printout of this calculation, giving a confidence level of 88 percent in the assumed failure rate of 0.1 percent per month.

Cumulative survival analysis successfully gives an unconditional standardized measure of past device reliability, based on unit exposure. The measure is the number of months before a target survival rate is reached.*

Random linear failure analysis will predict future performance based on past exposure, even though no failures have yet occurred. However, a necessary assumption is that failures, when they do occur, will be randomly and linearly scattered.

NOTES

1. Berkson et al., "Calculation of Survival Rates of Cancer Patients." *Proc. Staff Meetings, Mayo Clinic* 25 (1950): 270.

2. A. Schaudig et al., "Comparison of Function Time of Different Pacemaker Systems." *Ann. Cardiol.* 20, no. 4 (1971): 357.

3. G. Green, "Progress in Pacemaker Technology." *J. Electrocardiol.* 7, no. 4 (1974): 375.

4. A. Schaudig et al., "Comparison of Function Time of Different Pacemaker Systems."

5. V. Parsonnet, S. Furman, and N. Smyth, "Implantable Cardiac Pacemakers: Status Report and Resource Guideline (ICHD)." *Circulation* 50 (1974): A21.

6. D. Rosenbaum et al., *USAEC Statistical Guideline for Device Testing*. 1973.

---

*This method is currently in use in both the Cardiac Data Corp. reports and in the "Performance of Cardiac Pacemaker Pulse Generators" reports by Billitch et al. that appear in *PACE*.

6

STERILIZATION

STERILIZATION OF IMPLANTABLE DEVICES

Five methods which have been used for sterilization of implantable devices are: 1)cold chemical sterilization; 2) radiation; 3)ethylene oxide gas (ETO); 4) steam; and 5) 150°C dry heat.

Cold Chemical Sterilization

All our first implants were sterilized by immersion in bactericidal fluids. We used zephiran, Bard-Parker solution, Clorox, "Amerse," and other germicidal solutions. Some were very corrosive and the device had to be carefully rinsed in sterile water or sterile saline before implant. J. Boretos points out that cold chemical sterilization can leave an electrically conductive coating on component surfaces that could form unwanted short-circuit paths.[1] None of the cold chemical sterilization methods were 100 percent effective. We see no reason to use any of them today.

Radiation

Sterilization by X-ray, gamma ray, or nuclear radiation is too expensive a method to see widespread use in most hospitals. The capital cost for the equipment far exceeds that of the steam autoclave or the ETO gas sterilizer. However, radiation sterilization is seeing increasing use for sterilizing soft materials outside the hospital area. It has one particular advantage in that sealed and packaged materials may be sterilized in their shipping containers. We have made considerable use of this type of sterilization with our plastic containers for cloning plants. These containers will not withstand autoclave temperatures. Even very small amounts of residual ETO gas would be toxic to the plants. With radiation sterilization, unopened shipments of plastic containers can be processed in their containers and opened only in our sterile, tissue culture laboratory. However, devices having metal components will shield the radiation and prevent proper sterilization of some parts of the device. Thus, except for its expense, radiation sterilization is useful for bandages, plastics, and soft materials in the hospital, but is not generally used for implantable prosthetics. However, the Association for Advancement of Medical Instrumentation had, in draft,[2] a proposed recommended practice for radiation sterilization.

In 1980, we were involved in instrumentation for engine controls for a proposed nuclear powered aircraft. Transistor controls, although very new at the time, were felt be be needed because of the severe vibrational environment. We were, of course, greatly concerned about nuclear damage to electronic devices. Our investigation revealed that the critical component is the semiconductor and that the damage level is about 10^{13} NVT (neutrons versus time) or 10^7 roentgens. This is far above the lethal level for humans, so we subsequently had no concern about clinical therapeutic radiation effects on pacemakers.

More recently it was discovered that therapeutic radiation was having a deleterious effect on clinically implanted pacemakers using integrated circuits. The culprit was found to be the MOSFET transistor chip. The situation was serious enough for Seymour Furman[3] to organize a series of four papers from three countries into a symposium on the problem. Pulse generator failure was clinically documented with accumulated radiation of as little as 3×10^3 rads, over three orders of magnitude less than with older junction transistor devices.

Thus radiation sterilization of active implantable devices should probably not be considered.

Ethylene Oxide Gas Sterilization

Ethylene oxide gas (ETO) sterilization is becoming the principal means of sterilization in modern hospitals. It is the only means used by most suppliers of prosthetic devices. Some plastics such as silicone rubber actually absorb the gas and become sterilized in depth. ETO sterilizers operate at a maximum of about 135°F which is not high enough to damage even zinc-mercury batteries. Thus it has become commonly used for sterilizing pacemakers.

However, ETO has some drawbacks. The gas is extremely toxic. ETO sterilizers must be very carefully operated and very carefully maintained if they are to be safe. In 1983 OSHA considered reducing the permissible limits of ETO gas around sterilizers from 50 parts per million (ppm) to 1 ppm. Many users and manufacturers question whether such stringent limits can be routinely met, or even measured. OSHA formed an unlikely alliance with a labor organization and petitioned the Environmental Protection Agency (EPA) to limit the number of hours that operators would be permitted near ETO machines.

Monitoring of the work area for ETO contamination is recognized as a necessity. M. Reichart has reported a dual monitoring system to check such environments in a hospital.[4] For routine measurements, a semiconductor sensor is used. However, this sensor also responds to substances such as isopropyl alcohol, so a more complex infrared spectrometer is periodically used as a backup. An alternative is individual gas sampling monitors carried by each operator with subsequent laboratory analysis of the samples. Reichart finds this method costly, and also says that it supplies warning information too late to alleviate a problem, should one occur.

Material sterilized with ETO must be thoroughly aerated before use since any residual gas will produce necrosis in tissue. J. Boretos suggests a seven-day aeration period for silicones and rubber.[5] He also points out that PVC materials previously sterilized with gamma radiation should not be resterilized with ETO since significant amounts of ethylene chlorohydrin could be formed. Rendall-Baker notes also that ETO is a solvent for polymethylmethacrylate.[6]

To us a major problem is the fact that ETO will not kill hepatitis pathogens. Thus it is an unacceptable sterilizer for prosthetics that are to be reused in another patient. With the increased cost of pacemakers, reuse is common in developing countries and is even being considered in the United States. We see no objections if the device can be confidently sterilized and all proteinacious material removed.

S. Laufman[7] and C. Bruch[8] both note the increasing call for quantification of sterilization procedures, rather than the "empirical overkill of the past." J. Murtaugh et al.[9] note that improper moisture preconditioning is another factor which can invalidate proper sterilization with ETO.

The Association for Advancement of Medical Instrumentation[10,11,12] has recognized the need for ETO standards with several proposed standards, guidelines, and recommended practices.

ETO gas has many advantages but it certainly is not the ideal sterilization method. We prefer steam sterilization and suggest that all medical devices should be manufactured to withstand steam autoclave temperatures.

Steam Sterilization

Steam autoclaving is the oldest and, in our opinion, the best means of sterilizing implantable prosthetic devices. It is simple. The equipment need be nothing more than a home food pressure cooker on a charcoal fire in a jungle hospital. Standard autoclaving subjects material to 250°F for twenty to thirty minutes. Flash autoclave goes to 270°F for five minutes.

For the first two decades of pacing, zinc-mercury batteries and then lithium iodine batteries precluded the autoclaving of pacemakers. Since pacemaker pulse generators could not be autoclaved anyway, circuit designers used smaller and less expensive low-temperature components. In the 1980s, however, several new battery designs emerged which were autoclavable. We think that now pacemaker designers should go back to their drawing boards and redesign their circuits to withstand 250°F. Achieving the autoclavable battery required a new design, but achieving autoclavable components is merely a matter of selection. The military has long specified 125°C components for many aerospace applications. In a previous chapter on pulse generators we showed a steam sterilizable pulse generator with a lithium silver vanadium oxide (SVO) battery. This pulse generator has been autoclaved fifteen times and has operated within specifications for seven days at 125°C.

Dry Heat Sterilization

Steam autoclaves and dry heat sterilizers operate on quite different principles. The steam autoclave kills bacteria by coagulating proteins. Dry heat sterilizers operate by oxidizing the bacteria at higher temperatures.

Few electronic components and few plastic materials will survive long at 150°C. Thus we have never seriously considered this means of sterilization. Interestingly enough, the battery, which limited sterilization temperatures of early pacemakers, is not the limiting factor here. One new battery design (lithium sulfuryl chloride) will operate continuously at 150°C.

The design of steam sterilizers is a mature art and is well documented by a number of accepted standards and guidelines.[13,14]

NOTES

1. J. Boretos, "Polymer Considerations for Implant Electronics." In *Medical Engineering* 5, no. 84, edited by Charles Ray (Chicago: Yearbook Publishers, 1974), 1120.

2. Association for Advancement of Medical Instrumentation (AAMI) Recommended Practice (Proposed), "Process Control Guidelines for Gamma Radiation Sterilization of Medical Devices," 1983.

3. S. Furman, "Radiation Effects on Implanted Devices." *PACE* 5, no. 2 (1982): 145.

4. M. Reichert, "Infection Control: Ethylene Oxide Environmental Monitoring in a Health Care Facility." *Med. Inst.* 17, no. 2 (1983): 113.

5. J. Boretos, "Polymer Considerations for Implant Electronics."

6. L. Rendall-Baker and R. Roberts, "Gas Versus Steam Sterilization." *Med.-Surg. Rev.* 4 (1969): 10.

7. S. Laufman, "Toward Improved Safety, Efficiency and Economy of Sterilization Procedures." *Med. Inst.* 17, no. 3 (1983): 203.

8. C. Bruch, "Guest Editorial." *Med. Inst.* 17, no. 3 (1983): 205.

9. J. Murtaugh and G. Whitaker, "Preconditioning for Moisture Control in Ethylene Oxide Sterilization." *Med. Inst.* 17, no. 3 (1983): 211.

10. AAMI Recommended Practice, "Guidelines for Industrial ETO Sterilization of Medical Devices," 1981.

11. AAMI Recommended Practice, "Good Hospital Practice: Ethylene Oxide Gas," 1981.

12. AAMI Technology Assessment Report, "Industrial Ethylene Oxide Sterilization of Medical Devices." TAR-1, 1983.

13. AAMI Recommended Practice, "Good Hospital Practice: Steam Sterilization and Sterility Assurance," 1980.

14. American National Standards Institute (ANSI)/AAMI Standard, "Hospital Steam Sterilizers." ST-8, 1983.

FOR FURTHER READING

AAMI Draft Standard (Preliminary Draft), "Standard for Ethylene Oxide Sterilizers for Use in Health Care Facilities," 1983.

AAMI Recommended Practice (Draft), "Guidelines for Determining ETO Residual Levels in Medical Devices," 1983.

7

MICROCALORIMETRY*

Microcalorimeters with the capability of detecting heat changes at microwatt levels have been described by P. Monk et al.,[1] S. Pennington,[2] and E. Prosen et al.[3] These devices have long been used in microbiology and in physical and nuclear chemistry to identify and quantify microreactions, but their existence was apparently not evident to battery chemists until recently. In the past the only method for the evaluation of the internal self-discharge characteristics of batteries was to store them for a long period and then to discharge them under controlled conditions. The difference between the capacity obtained for fresh batteries and that obtained for stored batteries would then be that capacity lost in storage through self-discharge. In most military/commercial high drain rate battery applications, self-discharge is only of secondary interest, but in an implantable cardiac pacemaker such self-discharge (at least in older aqueous battery systems) eventually amounts to 30 percent or more of the initial battery capacity. Furthermore, implantable batteries have design service lives of five to ten years. Thus the testing required to evaluate self-discharge by classical means cannot be completed until long after the battery design becomes obsolete.

During a visit to the Siemans Elema (now St. Jude's Medical) pacemaker laboratories in Stockholm in 1975, Haaken Elmqvist suggested to us the use of a microcalorimeter to evaluate internal self-discharge. Siemans (Germany) had used a small commercial microcalorimeter to make rough measurements on single small button cells, and A. Thoren

---

*Please refer to the appendix of this book for more information about microcalorimetry.

subsequently reported this work in Tokyo.[4] Two days later the same suggestion was made to us in Dieren, Netherlands, by Eichmans, president of Vitatron Corp., another pacemaker manufacturer.

We subsequently discussed the idea intensively with E. Prosen of the National Bureau of Standards and with Roger Hart of Tronac Inc. of Ogden, Utah. Prosen had designed several small microcalorimeters for the Bureau of Standards, and Hart had built a number of differential microcalorimeters for the University of Utah.

Coincident with these discussions we began construction of a microcalorimeter of the Prosen design, but with a much larger aperture to accommodate pacemaker batteries. Our first unit was completed and used in May 1976.[5]

DESIGN

The microcalorimeter consists of a tight-fitting capsule of high-conductivity (heat) metal (silver, copper, or aluminum) containing the test battery and surrounded by bismuth telluride heat flow sensors. These sensors are thermopiles very similar to those used in nuclear pacemakers to convert the heat of decaying Pu^{238} into electrical energy. The thermocouple banks are connected in series and produce about 0.2 uV for each microwatt of heat. An internal X1000 operational amplifier amplifies the signal to the millivolt level, after which the signal is then recorded on a standard strip chart recorder at a rate of 1cm per hour.

The thermopiles are all heat-sinked to a common massive aluminum block. This block is thermally insulated in a piece of 8-inch diameter, $\frac{3}{8}$-inch thick aluminum pipe, thermostatically held at 37 ±0.001°C. This assembly is thermally insulated in a larger 12-inch diameter piece of aluminum pipe. The whole device is air insulated within a plyboard box thermostatically held at 30 ±1°C. The temperature of the microcalorimeter laboratory itself is maintained at about 20 ±0.5°C.

OPERATION

Initially, several days are necessary to allow the empty microcalorimeter to attain thermal equilibrium. Insertion of a battery immediately produces an offscale transient thermal response that requires fifteen to thirty minutes to return on scale. The stabilization time also depends on the temperature of the battery at the time of insertion. This period can be as much as twenty-four hours and has two distinct time constants. The first is the

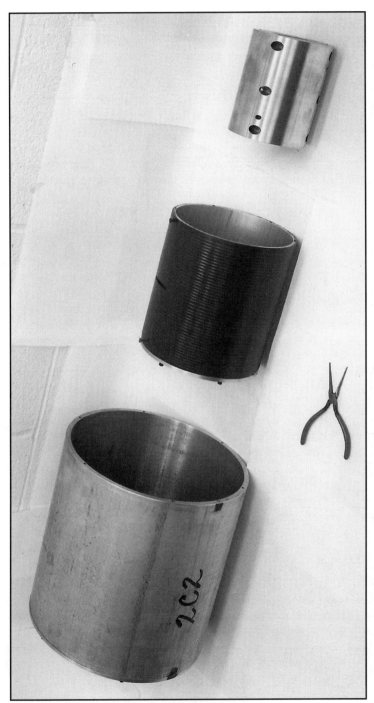

A disassembled microcalorimeter. From right to left: an aluminum block in which the thermopiles are heat-sinked, aluminum pipe thermostatically held at 37% ± 0.001° C, and a second 12-inch diameter aluminum pipe.

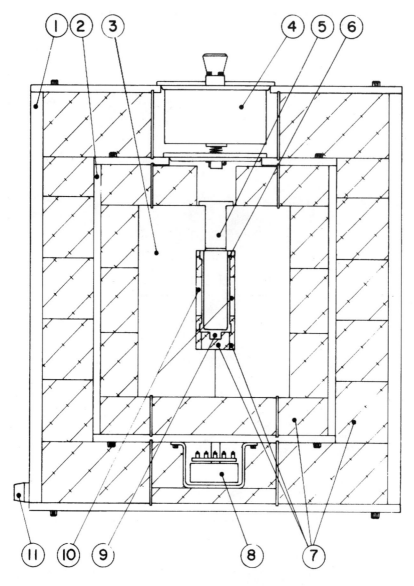

Microcalorimeter functional diagram. Parts list for functional diagram: 1. outer shell; 2. controlled shell; 3. heat sink; 4. cover assembly; 5. heat sink plug; 6. cell holder; 7. foamed polyurethane; 8. signal amplifier; 9. calibration resistor; 10. bismuth telluride sensors; 11. terminal strip.

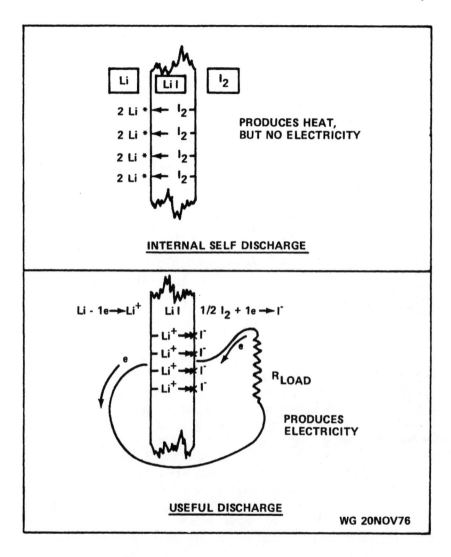

heat stabilization of the metal battery case (in direct contact with the inner metal capsule). This reaches equilibrium quickly, typically in less than an hour. The second time constant is much longer and seems to be dependent upon the much larger heat content of the lithium and iodine and the slow thermal transfer characteristics of the materials. By preheating the battery to as near 37°C as possible and quickly transferring it to the chamber, we have been able to reduce the insertion transient to four hours for rough work and to twelve hours for precise measurements.

Calibration is accomplished by passing a known current through very fine wires (low heat conductivity) to a precision resistor temporarily placed in the capsule. These wires are brought out through a tortuous helical path to minimize heat conduction. Precise measurement of voltage and time permit a very accurate determination of heat generated. This apparatus is capable of measuring the heat exotherm of a grain of germinating rice.

Numerous measurements on 22 WGLtd. Model 755 batteries (3.0 Ah) consistently gave readings of 37 ±17 (s.d.) microwatts. Some testing was also done on older WGLtd. Model 752 batteries (1.5 Ah) with the expectation of lower losses due to the lesser amounts of materials present. Surprisingly we observed an average value nearer 50 microwatts on these batteries. We then built a number of special battery enclosures containing only one component of the battery. One such enclosure contained three drops of epoxy, a component specific to the WGLtd. Model 752 battery. This epoxy was used to secure the plastic module in the metal case before welding. After insertion of the battery case into the microcalorimeter, the exotherm exhibited an increase to over 25 microwatts and took several hours to attain equilibrium. Obviously, we were observing the exotherm from the three drops of epoxy as the accelerated cure continued at the 37°C level.

We found much the same results but in varying degrees with curing polyester, the mix of poly-2-vinylpyridine with iodine in the cathode complex and in cyanoacrylate adhesive, all of which were used in this battery. Because the sum of these exotherms is probably ten times the true internal self-discharge of the battery, it is necessary to accurately detect and to quantify their magnitude and the dependence upon time. When this is done, these large numbers can be safely subtracted to arrive at the small, but important, value for the self-discharge.

It is also necessary to consider carefully every possible reaction, exothermic or endothermic, because one type will tend to cancel the heat of the other. At present we suspect that all reactions are exothermic.

EFFECT OF LOAD CURRENT ON SELF-DISCHARGE

In the process of testing two samples of a 1.5 Ah lithium iodine battery (WGLtd. Model 752) in our microcalorimeter, we found that adding an external load (outside the microcalorimeter) significantly lowered the heat generated by the battery. Further evaluation at different values of load confirmed that internal self-discharge was higher under open-circuit conditions and decreased as the current drain from the battery was increased.

As a result of these findings we theorize that self-discharge in solid-electrolyte lithium-iodine cells arises from migration of iodine molecules through the lithium iodide electrolyte toward the anode. At the lithium-lithium iodide interface, iodine probably combines with lithium to form lithium iodide, producing heat but no useful electrical current. This is in contrast to the normal battery reaction in which lithium yields an electron to the load and then freely migrates, in ionic form, through lithium iodide crystalline defects to the iodine complex. The iodide ion, having acquired an electron from the load, then combines to form additional lithium iodide. The lithium iodide solid electrolyte behaves somewhat as a molecular semiconductor with conduction through defects which emulate "molecular holes." The reaction is diffusion limited and will quickly lower the iodine concentration at the interface, reducing the self-discharge of the cell to insignificant levels. In addition, there is superim-

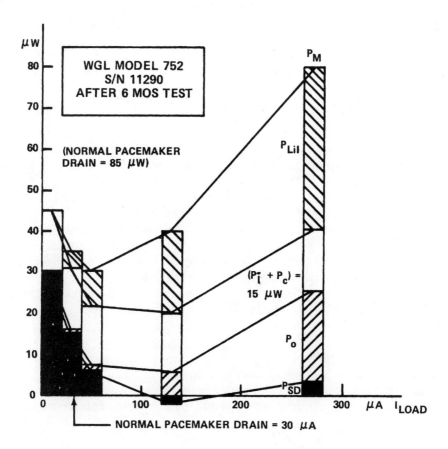

posed the effect of the increasing thickness of the electrolyte with continued discharge, further decreasing the internal discharge reaction.

There remain a number of other heat sources within the cell which may produce detectable heat. In addition to 1)P_{sd}, the chemical self-discharge reaction mentioned above, they are:

2) P_o		I^2R loss from load current flowing through internal ohmic resistances of the cell. $P_o = I_{load} (E_{oc} - E_{loaded})$.
3) P_i		Electronic leakage losses across marginal insulating materials.
4) P_{LiI}		The normal heat of formation of lithium iodide formed in the usual ionic manner (see calculation below).
5) P_c		Innocuous exotherm from continued curing of epoxy, polyester, and complexed materials, and so on.

P_o and P_{LiI} are calculable from direct measurements of I_{load}, Faraday's Law, and the knowledge of the thermodynamics relative to the formation of LiI. The remainder of the microcalorimeter reading consists of the sum of P_i, P_c, and P_{sd}. If we assume that P_{sd} approaches zero at high load currents, then $(P_i + P_c)$ can be measured. Since P_i and P_c should not be a function of load current then the remaining power at more normal load currents should be P_{sd}:

$$P_{sd} = P_{tot} - (P_o + P_i + P_{LiI} + P_c)$$

Our microcalorimeter, like that of Prosen, was a single-ended device that made an absolute measurement of heat flow. More recently Roger Hart has designed a differential device, manufactured by Tronac Corp. This device, because of its differential nature, is much more stable than ours, and we do most of our work with one or more of his devices.

We find ourselves relying more heavily each day on what our microcalorimeters tell us. We no longer undertake destructive analysis of a failed battery without first measuring its heat output. We make monthly measurements of all prototypes of new designs. We see a larger version of the microcalorimeter as indispensable in future pacemaker evaluation, both for prototype testing and for failure analysis.

CONCLUSIONS

Presently available microcalorimeters easily demonstrate a reduction in noise to the one microwatt level and enlargement of the test aperture to accommodate larger batteries as well as complete pacemaker pulse generators. Successful operation at the one microwatt noise level should permit wide application into the study of internal self-discharge in batteries, corrosion processes on pipelines, orthopedic structures, and, in fact, on any well defined exothermic or endothermic process. The value of microcalorimetry testing was recently demonstrated to us when a CPI lithium-powered pacemaker with a WGLtd. Model 702E battery was removed from an Australian patient, still operative, after twenty-two years of service.

NOTES

1. P. Monk et al., *Acta. Chim. Scand.* 22 (1968): 1842.
2. S. Pennington et al., *Analytical Biochem.* 32 (1969): 251.
3. E. Prosen, "Microcalorimetry Applied to Biochemical Processes." In *Thermal Analysis: Comparative Studies on Materials*, edited by Kambe and Garn. (New York: Wiley, 1974), 253.
4. A. Thoren et al., "Test Results for Long-life Batteries for Cardiac Pacemakers." *Proc. 5th Intl. Symp. on Cardiac Pacing*, Tokyo, 1976.
5. W. Holmes et al., "A Microcalorimeter for Nondestructive Analysis of Pacemakers and Pacemaker Batteries." *Proc. 28th Power Sources Symposium*, Atlantic City, 1977: 226.

FOR FURTHER READING

Unterecker, D., "The Use of a Microcalorimeter for Analysis of Load-dependent Processes Occurring in a Primary Battery." *J. Electrochem.* 125, no. 12 (1978): 1907.

Untereker and Boone, *Proc. NBS Cardiac Pacemaker Workshop*, Washington, D.C., 1978.

8

ELECTRONIC CONTROL
OF GROWTH

OSTEOGENESIS

It has long been known that mechanical bending of a long bone will produce osteogenesis on the concave side. Over three decades ago, I. Yasuda in Japan attributed this to piezoelectric potential and reported acceleration of bone growth by application of electrical stimuli.[1] This information was available only in Japanese and was not reported in the West. A decade later C. Bassett in New York observed that the normal long bones have a negative potential at the ends where growth occurs, but have a positive potential at the center.[2] Should such a bone be broken, the potential at the break will go strongly negative and healing will commence. Bassett suggested that if negativity is accompanied by healing, one should be able to electrically stimulate the area of the break with cathodic current and accelerate healing. He did this and reported positive results.[3] Subsequently C. Brighton in Philadelphia performed similar experiments using negatively driven percutaneous stainless steel needles residing invasively in the break area.[4] Later R. Becker, who originally worked with Bassett, reported achievement of osteogenesis with active devices, totally implanted.[5]

None of the above investigators was able to prove a mechanism for electro-osteogenesis. Yasuda theorized that the piezoelectric potential produced a negatively charged area, causing the osteogenesis.[6] He later used an electret to create an osteogenic current of only 10^{-24} amperes which he felt was sufficient.[7] An electret is a Teflon pellet which is placed between two metal plates, charged to 5,000 volts, heated to softening, and then allowed to cool while still in the high-voltage field. This freezes the dipoles in an aligned position and produces a permanent static charge on the Teflon tape. An electret is the electrostatic equivalent of a permanent magnet. When placed in physiological saline, Na^+ and Cl^- ions will rush around the pellet to balance the electret charge. During the life of the electret, a charge element will discharge, releasing a salt ion which will rush around the pellet to restore the balance. This results in a very small ionic current of about 10^{-24} amperes which Yasuda felt was sufficient to trigger osteogenesis. Becker stated that a current of a fraction of a microampere was optimal,[8] while Brighton used 80 uA divided among four electrodes.[9]

To an electrical engineer, it is quite surprising to see such a wide range of current levels declared to be optimal. Either the actual current level is immaterial or a number of different but equally effective mechanisms must be at work. We feel that the actual mechanism or mechanisms of osteogenesis must be discovered before such variances in data can be understood.

Geoffrey Wickham in Australia built total osteogenic implants similar to those of Becker but with a higher output current, nearer 10 mA.[10] In the meantime, Bassett, in an attempt to achieve a noninvasive procedure, had begun using a pulsed magnetic field with the bone defect positioned between two toroidal air-core coils.[11] Watson in England extended this principle to the utilization of somewhat smaller and more efficient iron-core coils.[12]

Of the above systems, three had achieved FDA approval by 1983: Basset's pulsed electromagnetic field (PEMF) device, manufactured by Electro Devices Inc. in New Jersey; Brighton's transcutaneous stainless steel electrically-driven wires, manufactured by Zimmer Inc. in Warsaw, Indiana; and Wickham's active implant, manufactured by Telectronics Pty. Ltd. in Australia. None of these investigators claimed 100 percent success and none was able to explain (at least to our satisfaction) what mechanism was involved in successful treatment, or why treatment sometimes failed. At best, the major investigators claim only that their systems have a success rate at least equal to surgical intervention (pinning, plating, and so on) at a far lower cost.

SO WHAT MAKES IT WORK?

L. Norton et al. attributed osteogenesis to modulation of cyclic AMP and believes this may be the intracellular signal derived from the extracellular electrical stimulation.[13] C. Brighton suggests that the electrical field modifies the pH of the defect area, encouraging osteogenesis.[14] D. Knighton et al. have performed some interesting experiments on monomolecular membrane growth across a plastic insert in a rabbit's ear. He presents strong evidence that revascularization (which is directly correlated with osteogenesis) is a function of pO_2 gradient. Following is a complete abstract of one of Knighton's recent papers.

Interrelationship between pO_2, vascularity and tissue regeneration.

D.R. Knighton, M.D., and T.K. Hunt, M.D. Department of Surgery, University of California, San Francisco.

Angiogenesis, the directed proliferation of capillary endothelium, is a prominent feature of both soft tissue and bone healing. In both situations the reparative process proceeds from the well-oxygenated, perfused edge of the wound or fracture toward the central hypoxic dead space until that dead space is filled with perfused, normaxic connective tissue and/or bone.

Recent experiments in soft tissue wound healing and angiogenesis show that oxygen gradients from the perfused edge of the healing wound toward the hypoxic dead space are necessary for the induction of angiogenesis and subsequent healing. Using a modification of Clark's rabbit ear chamber the pO_2 of the wound space was manipulated by placing either oxygen-permeable or -impermeable coverslips over the chamber. Oxygen-permeable coverslips allowed the normally hypoxic dead space to equilibrate with atmospheric oxygen, thus raising the pO_2 from its normally low range of 2–10 mm Hg to approximately 150. Impermeable coverslips kept the healing chamber at its normally low pO_2. By arranging the coverslips so that an impermeable cover was above a permeable cover, the pO_2 in the healing chamber could be raised or lowered at any time in the healing process.

When oxygen-impermeable coverslips were left in place throughout the experiment, healing progressed in an orderly fashion until the healing chamber was filled with new capillaries and connective tissue. Oxygen-permeable covers used from time of implantation eliminated new capillary growth into the chamber and totally suppressed the normal healing response. When the oxygen gradient was obliterated by removing the oxygen-impermeable cover at various stages in the healing process, capillary growth stopped and in some cases receded, leaving a "doughnut" of new capillaries with a hole in the center. If the gradient was destroyed and then reestablished by removing and then replacing the impermeable cover, angiogenesis continued, but at a slower rate than when the oxygen gradient was in place from the beginning of the experiment.

Implantation of metallic electrodes into soft tissue, the medullary canal of a long bone, or a nonunited fracture site also produces local oxygen gradients similar to those present in a soft tissue wound.

Oxygen diffuses poorly through connective tissue. Therefore, the presence of an inert metal rod in vascularized tissue will create a local hypoxic oxygen gradient from the nearest perfused capillary to the rod. These gradients have been measured by Silver using microelectrodes. When a current is applied to the electrode the anode consumes oxygen, thus steepening the oxygen gradient. This artificially produced hypoxic gradient creates a local environment similar to an incised wound in soft tissue or a fracture, and results in a proliferative response from the surrounding connective tissue.

The cellular and biochemical signals which initiate and regulate wound repair, fracture repair, and electrically induced bone and soft tissue proliferation are still poorly understood. Perhaps the presence of a local hypoxic gradient, a common aspect of all these physiologic processes, is one of the regulatory mechanisms which initiate and sustain the healing process. The hypoxic focus could theoretically influence the production of "growth factors" from inflammatory cells in the wound or fracture site, and/or potentiate proliferation and differentiation of effector cells.[15]

Since three osteogenic devices were at one time approved by the FDA and were in rather extensive use, we must be receptive to the idea that they work. However, our own results have been less than remarkable. We would feel more confidence if a proven theory existed, explaining their function.

We performed three sets of experiments with total implants, all of which were interesting, but all were inconclusive. For this reason we have never reported our results in the technical literature. Thus, the work presented here is unpublished.

1. We supplied some miniature implant devices to J. Spadero's group at Syracuse, New York, in support of a previous program which had used devices made by others.[16] We used a single field-effect transistor, powered by a silver mercury hearing-aid battery. The total device weighed under 3g. It delivered a constant-current of 10 nA ±5 percent into any load from zero to 1 megohm. Some units were supplied in other current ratings. The electrode lead was a 0.010"D silver 10 percent palladium wire, wound on a 0.010"D mandril, resulting in a very flaccid 0.030"D helical spring coil, which was then sheathed in silicone rubber tubing. The lead terminated in a 2cm length of single, bare wire. Alloying the silver with palladium raised its tensile strength over five times, to over 100,000 psi, without compromising its polarization properties. The anode was a 2-turn helix of 0.020"D pure silver. The cathode electrode is described in more detail in chapter 3 on electrodes.

Stimulators were implanted in a number of white Swiss mice with the 2 cm of exposed wire inserted in the medulary canal (a canal in the

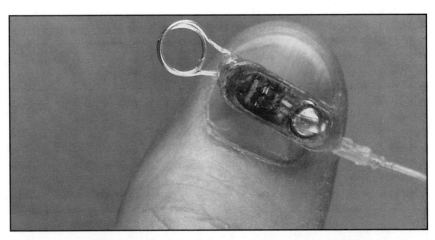

Osteogenic stimulators used in mice.

bone marrow). We were unable to duplicate results previously obtained. Our stimulators had very flaccid, spring-coil electrodes. The previously used stimulators had stiff, relatively heavy stainless steel wires which may have contributed to the osteogenesis that we failed to obtain.

2. Dr. N. C. Rath at State University of New York at Buffalo (SUNYAB), Department of Biophysics, had done some work[17] after A. Reddi[18] in which demineralized bone was powdered, filled into dissolvable capsules, and then implanted in the abdomens of rats. We built a number of stimulators with silver-palladium cathode wires extending through the capsule, delivering a cathodic current of 1 uA to the bone powder pellets. In the past, such experiments provided a well-controlled method of testing for osteogenesis in various preparations in a single-animal environment without sacrificing the animal. We implanted some capsules with stimulators and some without. In some cases, we saw more osteogenesis on stimulated capsules than on unstimulated controls, but our results were inconsistent. Unfortunately, Dr. Rath left the university at this time for a position in another city and we did not continue our work. We were sorry to drop this work because this model seemed to us to present a uniquely well controlled environment, with both experiment and control in the same nonexpendable animal.

3. In a final experiment, at the SUNYAB Department of Orthopedics we produced standard defects in a number of canine legs after J. Medige under Dr. Eugene Mindel.[19] A cylinder was excised from the femur of a dog and replaced with a cylindrical silicone plug. Over a period of weeks the size of the femur near the defect would thicken markedly. After a period of eight weeks, the animal was sacrificed and the femur recov-

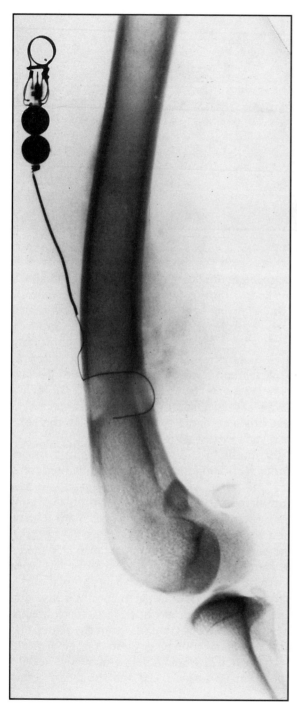

Osteogenic stimulator implanted with electrode in a cylindrical defect in a dog's femur, after Medige (1982).

THE WAY IT WAS

A few years ago I had an opportunity to visit Findhorn, an "alternate" agricultural communal society on the north coast of Scotland, near Inverness. The Findhorn people insist that plants have souls that respond to loving kindness with fantastic growth, including fifty-pound cabbages and fist-sized strawberries. The community exuded peace, contentment, and love. I was much impressed. On my return home, I sat down in my bean patch and talked to the beans. They responded affirmatively, nodding their heads and we all felt great. But they didn't grow any faster. I guess it didn't really do much for the beans, but it probably did me a lot of good.

---

ered. The defect was examined and the femur was stressed to failure in a calibrated testing machine built by Dr. Medige, a mechanical engineer.

We built a number of stimulators similar to those previously described. The wire cathode was inserted between the silicon plug and the bone, within the defect, in a number of animals, with an equal number being left as controls. We saw some acceleration of bone growth in stimulated animals, but not enough to be statistically significant. If one old and somewhat sick animal were removed from the study, then the results became marginally significant, but we did not feel such manipulation of data was necessary.

ACCELERATION OF GROWTH OF SOFT TISSUE

M. Mosharaffa has suggested using cathodic current to accelerate the fixation of endocardial electrodes.[20] One of his electrode designs includes a screen tip surface enclosing a platinum mesh. The assembly is designed to present a maximum of metal/fluid interface area, to minimize the interface impedance to stimulation current. Mosharaffa's suggestion would involve an initial cathodic DC current of perhaps 10 to 100 nA for perhaps a week to accelerate the ingrowth of endocardial tissue into the screened cavity. If the mechanism of osteogenesis becomes known, perhaps this knowledge can be extrapolated to soft tissue.

B. Harrison et al. has reported a pronounced effect of cathodic stimulation of 100 nA DC on the regeneration of damaged nerves.[21] The electric field tended to arrest the degradation of the damaged nerve and thus considerably speeded up its regeneration.

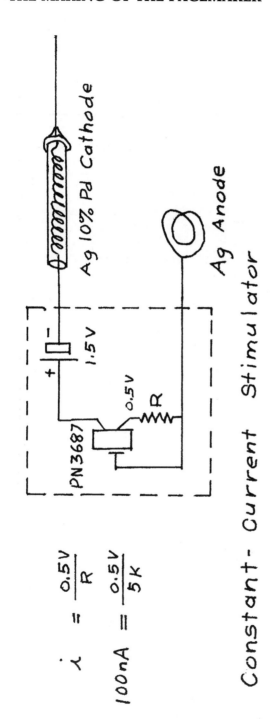

Constant-current stimulator.

ACCELERATION OF GROWTH OF PLANT TISSUE

One occasionally finds in the literature references to speeding up the growth of plants by electrical stimulation. Much of it must be relegated to the same category as "plant music" recordings that contain soothing rhythms with no percussion. The playing of such recordings supposedly benefits the growth of plants.

However, some serious work has been done on plant stimulation.

D. Jones et al. in Germany reported significant improvement of differentiation in bean and potato suspension cultures (clones, grown in test tubes) over controls grown without stimulation.[22] They used a pulsed magnetic field with single pulses at 15 Hz for six hours on, followed by six hours off. Controls and test samples were grown in the same container, but with the magnetic field shielded from the control.

Jorge Reynolds in Bogota, Colombia, was experimenting with the effect of electric fields in accelerating the growth of fruit trees, but had no definitive data as of late 1983.[23] Ginsler in Tucson, Arizona, reported acceleration of plant growth by introducing DC currents into the soil.[24]

In summary, electrical acceleration of growth is probably the most poorly understood subject of any we have discussed in these twelve chapters. Much of the reported work is anecdotal, little of it is repeatable, and there is very little understanding of any of the basic mechanisms involved, plant or animal. However, it remains a fascinating field with fantastic rewards to both investigator and society for any advances in understanding and application that can be achieved. We consider this to be a most difficult and complex field whose challenges should not be underestimated. But that only makes it more interesting. We must keep an open mind, even to Findhorn*, although I do not think the scientific answers will be found there.

NOTES

1. I. Yasuda, "Piezoelectricity of Bone." *I Kyota Med Soc.* 4 (1953): 395.

2. C. Bassett and R. Becker, "Generation of Electric Potentials in Bone in Response to Mechanical Stress." *Science* 137 (1962): 1063.

3. C. Bassett, "Electric Effects in Bone." *Scientific American* 213 (1965): 18.

4. C. Brighton, S. Adler, J. Black, N. Itada, and A. Friedenberg, "Cathodic Oxygen Consumption and Electrically Induced Osteogenesis." *Clin. Orthop.* 107 (1975): 277.

---

*The Scottish community referred to earlier in the chapter.

5. R. Becker, J. Spadero, and A. Marino, "Clinical Experiences with Low Intensity Direct Stimulation." *Clin. Orthop.* 124 (1977): 75.

6. I. Yasuda, "Piezoelectricity of Bone," 395.

7. I. Yasuda, "Electrical Callus and Callus Formation By Electret." *Clin. Orthop.* 124(1977): 53.

8. R. Becker et al., "Clinical Experiences with Low Intensity Direct Stimulation," 75.

9. C. Brighton, A. Friedenberg, E. Mitchell, and R. Bath, "Treatment of Non-union with Constant Direct Current." *Clin. Orthop.* 124 (1977): 106.

10. G. Wickham and F. Dwyer, "Bone Prosthesis." U.S. Patent 3,964,473, 1976.

11. C. Bassett, "Electric Effects in Bone," 18.

12. J. Watson and G. Downes, "Clinical Aspects of Bone Healing Using Electrical Phenomena." *Med. and Biol. Engin.* 17 (1979): 161.

13. L. Norton, G. Roday, and C. Bourret, "Epiphyseal Cartilage cAMP Changes Produced By Electrical and Mechanical Perturbation." *Clin. Orthop.* 124:59 (1977)

14. C. Brighton et al., "Treatment of Non-union with Constant Direct Current," 106.

15. D. Knighton and T. Hunt, "Interrelationship Between pO_2 Vascularity and Tissue Regeneration." *Trans. 17th Annual AAMI Meeting*, San Francisco, VI (1982): 62.

16. F. Ellis and S. Andrews, "Method of In-vivo Sterilization of Surgical Implantables." U.S. Patent 4,027,393, filed 1975, issued 1977.

17. N. Rath and A. Reddi, "Changes in Ornithine Decerbolase Activity During Matrix-induced Cartilage, Bone and Bone Marrow Differentiation." *Biochemical and Biophysical Research Communications* 81, no. 1 (New York: Academic Press, 1978), 106.

18. A. Reddi, "Collagen and Cell Differentiation." In *Biochemistry of Collagen 9*, edited by G. N. Ramachandron and A. H. Reddi (New York: Plenum Publishing Co., 1976), 449.

19. J. Medige, E. Mindell, and T. Doolittle, "Remodeling of Large Persistent Bone Defects." *Clin. Orthop.* 169 (1982): 275.

20. M. Mosharaffa, Personal communication, 1981.

21. B. Harrison, D. Haynes, and E. Weber, "The Effects of Electrical Stimulation on Peripheral Nerve Regeneration." *Trans 3rd Annual Meeting BRAGS*, San Francisco, III (1983): 18.

22. D. Jones and P. Bolwell, "The Effect of PEMF on In-vitro Differentiation of Bean and Potato Suspension Culture." *Trans. 3rd Annual Metting BRAGS*, San Francisco, III (1983): 40.

23. J. Reynolds, Personal communication, 1983.

24. Ginsler, Personal communication, 1979.

FOR FURTHER READING

Becker, R., "The Bioelectric Factors in Amphibian Limb Regeneration." *J. Bone, Joint Surgery* 43A (1961): 643.

Becker, R., and J. Spadero, "Electrical Stimulation of Partial Limb Regeneration in Mammals." *Bull. NY Acad. Med.* 48 (1972): 127.

Brighton, C., and S. Pollack, "Treatment of Non-union with a Capacitively Coupled Electrical Field: Preliminary Findings." *Trans. 3rd Annual Meeting BRAGS*, San Francisco III (1983): 1.

Brighton, C., Z. Friedenberg, and W. Redka, "Constant Current Power Pack for Bone Healing and Method of Use." U.S. Patent 3,842,841, filed 1971, issued 1974.

Deitch, E., A. Marino, V. Malaknok, and J. Albright, "Electrical Augmentation of Antibacterial Activity of Silver Ions." *Trans 3rd Annual Meeting BRAGS*, San Francisco III (1983): 59.

Duarte, L., "The Use of Ultrasound to Stimulate Non-union Healing." *Trans. 3rd Annual meeting BRAGS*, San Francisco, III (1983): 31.

Marino, A., V. Malaknok, E. Deitch, and J. Albright, "Electrical Properties of Silver Nylon." *Trans 3rd Annual Meeting BRAGS*, San Francisco, III (1983): 36.

Murray, J., and M. Lacy, "Pulsing Electromagnetic Fields Can Modulate the Production of Degraditive Enzymes By Synovial Cells." *Trans 3rd Annual Meeting BRAGS*, San Francisco, III (1983): 7.

Paterson, D., and R. Simonis, "Electrical Stimulation in the Treatment of Pseudoarthrosis of the Tibia." *Trans. 3rd Annual Meeting BRAGS*, San Francisco, III (1983): 2.

Spadero, J., T. Berger, S. Barranco, S. Chapin, and R. Becker, "Antibacterial Effects of Silver Electrodes with Weak Current." *Antibacterial Agents and Chemotherapy*: 637 (1974).

Spadero, J., D. Webster, and S. Chase, "Direct Current Activation of Bacteriostatic Silver Electrodes." *Trans. 3rd Annual Meeting BRAGS*, San Francisco, III (1983): 37.

9

ELECTRONIC CONTROL OF INFECTION

THE GERMICIDAL EFFECT OF SILVER IONS

Silver has long been used as an infection control agent. I painfully remember from childhood days my mother's administration of argerol for nasal congestion. Silver ointments have long been used in the treatment of burns, and silver nitrate drops were once used to counter infection in the eyes of newborn infants. Thus it is not surprising that several research groups have sought new ways to use silver ions for infection control. We would like to address ourselves here to the apparatus and methods for creating a much higher concentration of silver ions than that of the equilibrium state in saline solution.

Much of our early work had been done with R. Becker and J. Spadero of the Orthopedic Research Laboratory of the Veterans Administration Hospital at Syracuse, New York, but our own participation in this work is far from a success story. Perhaps the best introduction would be to copy verbatim from my 1979 research notebook #5, pp. 30–36:

THE WAY IT WAS

August 28, 1979
Joe Spadero had written several papers on electrically killing bacteria with positive current on anodes. He had demonstrated germicidal effects down to 40 nanoamperes, but had not had the

(continued)

---

funding to go lower. I wanted to look at this but had no way to prepare and incubate the cultures.

I talked to Janine Torba, a science teacher at the local high school, and she agreed to do some of the experiments in her AP (advance placement) biology class. I made up a number of Petri dishes with four to six holes around the periphery, drilled either with the WGLtd. CO_2 laser or with a butane microtorch. I mounted several pure silver anodes and common cathode (pure silver) in the holes. I insulated the wires with silicone tubing and sealed them in with medical adhesive. The common cathode was a helix of 0.020"D pure silver wire, about 10cm long, wound in a 2 to 3 cm D helix. The anodes were all 0.010"D pure silver with about 2cm of wire exposed beyond the end of the silicone tubing. The resistors were selected to give a range of currents from 25 nA (25 x 10^{-9}A) to 10uA. Torba and her class autoclaved my Petri dishes, filled them 5mm deep with sterile agar medium, and inoculated the medium with *Micrococcus luteus* (a laboratory bacteria). In twenty-four hours the bacteria had grown into colonies occluding the whole media. We applied current to some plates, starting after twenty-four hours, when bacterial growth was well advanced. Clear areas developed around all the stimulated anodes, but not around the unstimulated anodes. We then applied current to other new plates immediately upon inoculation. The areas near the stimulated anodes remained clear, but areas around unstimulated anodes became cloudy with bacterial growth, as did the rest of the plate. We washed out the media from old plates and replaced it with new media, but retained the old wires. Old wires which had been stimulated in the old plate, but left unstimulated in the new plate, still gave a marginal clearing effect. We concluded that the germicidal effect was indeed due to Ag^+ ion. No Ag^+ ion was generated in the vicinity of new unstimulated anodes but enough residual Ag^+ ion remained on previously stimulated anodes to assure some vestigial germicidal effect in anodes in reused plates, even though no stimulation was applied in the reuse.

The area of bacterial inhibition was limited to ±10mm from the wire, usually to ±5mm. Optimum clearing seemed to occur at about 100nA. Below that we got a more or less linear decrease in cleared area down to 25nA which was as low as we went. Above 100 nA we got little appreciable increase in cleared area. A ten-times increase in current gave only perhaps 10 percent more cleared area. We concluded that the Ag^+ ion is available, from anodically corroding metallic silver, at a much greater concentration than one sees from the dissociation of common silver salts such as AgCl or metallic Ag. ($AgNO_3$ and AgF are much more sol-

(continued)

uble but are also quite toxic). A century of literature has proved the ger-micidal effect of silver metal and silver salts in wound healing and so on, but the very low ionic concentration may have held its effect to such a low value that silver therapy has gradually fallen into disuse. No one thought of electrically corroding it until the work of Becker and Spadero. In 1983 they used electrically corroding silver wires for exper-imentally killing bacteria in osteomyelitis (inflammation of the bone marrow and adjacent bone) and corroding silver-nylon cloth for infec-tion control in tissue surrounding osteomyelitic bone.

We subsequently took some of our Petri dishes to Grand Island Bio-logical Co. (GIBCO), to Dr. Don Tartock and Dave Tricoli. They manu-facture nutrient media for growing tissue samples of plants and animals. Tiny samples were placed in a high-nutrient media which suppresses the normal tendency of the plant sample to grow roots and leaves. Instead the cells divide into colonies. When a colony is placed in another media with growth hormones, leaves and roots develop. Such a propagation method is perhaps most accurately termed "tissue culture" but might also come under a broad definition of "cloning." If one can find a non-infected leaf or root nodule on an infected parent plant, one might get a noninfected daughter clone. If, however, the parent has a systemic infection, then the clone, too, will be infected. Tricoli placed samples from a known infected *ficus elastica* (rubber plant) on the silver anodes of our plates and applied various currents to them for various times. His results were mixed, but in a number of samples run at about 1.0uaDC, he was able to get a clean daughter from a plant that had never pro-duced clean daughters by any means at his disposal.

There are important economic implications here: 1) The concept of tissue culture may well make greenhouses obsolete, except to harden off the new young shoots. The life cycle is about one month before ten new clones can be taken from a plant. Every six months, a single clone should produce one million offspring! If each is placed on an anodically stimu-lated silver loop, then each should be free from infection, even if its parent was infected. 2) An advantage of cloning is that each daughter will be genetically identical with its parent, same color, same smell, same taste, and so on. This could revolutionize the horticultural industry.

Dr. Kenneth Horst at Cornell University has been heavily involved with viroid research.[1] Viroids are the smallest known pathogen, one hun-dred times smaller than a virus. The first viroid was found in 1971 by Dr. L. Diener, a Swiss researcher working at the U.S. Department of Agricul-ture. Viroids consist of pure, naked RNA or DNA molecules encased in a

(continued)

protein sheath. The sheath enables the virus to generate antibodies which attach to the protein sheath and then are able to attack and kill the virus. Since the viroid has no protein sheath, and thus does not generate antibodies, it is most difficult to kill. Viroids can be boiled twelve minutes without damage!

We supplied Horst with a couple of our plates and he grew some plants in them, including chrysanthemums known to be infected with "chrysanthemum stunt," one of the plant viroids. Horst left the current (about 1uA) on for two weeks. (I told him only four hours!) The chrysanthemum survived. After two weeks, he ground up the plant and put it into a gel column. He then put 20v across the column (gel electrophoresis), causing the electromobile elements to migrate along the length of the column. The viroid should have migrated to a precise band, but after two weeks, no band was there. Horst said the sample was too small, and that such experiments sometimes don't work and need to be repeated. Nothing was conclusive, but still no viroid was detectable. That was enough for me, and I filed a patent application on it.[2]

Spadero did some work on floating tumor cells and killed them. I keep wondering if Ag^+ therapy wouldn't do something for leukemia. Elmer Erb, an old friend, is dying from this. If Ag^+ will preferentially kill leukemia cells, one might put an implant with an anodically corroding silver wire in a large vein. The body's circulatory system would get around the slow migration we see in the agar plate.

This 1979 entry in my research notebook summarizes what we had done to that point in time. We subsequently contacted the Cornell University potato research station in Lake Placid. They said they were trying to keep rid of viruses and viroids and didn't want us to bring any within a hundred miles of the place. Seems like a narrow-minded response, but I guess it all depends where you are coming from.

The following seven examples are taken from my work of 1981.[3]

Example I

Three identical arrangements of apparatus were set up to the foregoing description. The holes or apertures in the Pyrex test tubes were made by piercing the tubes with a butane touch. Silver wires were inserted through the holes in each of the tubes, and the protective tubes or sleeves were of silicone rubber. The protective tubes were sealed to the glass test tubes with Dow Corning type "A" medical adhesive. The silver wires defining the cathodes in each arrangement had a diameter of 0.02

inch and were formed into the bottom of each test tube in a single loop. The silver wires defining the anodes in each arrangement had a diameter of 0.01 inch and were brought to the center of each test tube and terminated in a small loop. The battery voltage was 6.0 volts and the resistor magnitude 2.7 megohms.

Each apparatus arrangement was sterilized in a steam autoclave, and then a nutrient medium was introduced into each test tube in an amount sufficient to cover the anode loop. The nutrient medium was Murashiga shoot multiplication medium A available from Grand Island Biological Co. under the number 500–119. A microscopic sample of *ficus elastica* (rubber plant) was infected with a gram negative bacteria and placed on the anode loop. The electrical current into the anode wire was approximately 2 microamperes d.c.

Previous preparations without the foregoing electronic excitation had shown overnight growth of bacterial colonies about the clone. The three examples with electronic excitation showed no bacterial clouds. Their growth continued on to produce disease-free plants. The foregoing evidences laboratory production of disease-free offspring from infected plant stock by the method and apparatus of the present invention.

Example II

The procedure of Example I was repeated, using one millimeter of leaf tissue taken from a *ficus elastica* known to be infected by an unknown bacteria. All previous attempts to get an uninfected clone from this parent had failed. The clone was placed in the nutrient solution resting on the anode loop of the pure silver wire. About one microampere of positive current was delivered to the anode for twenty-four hours. On repeated tests, currents ranging from 0.1 to 10 microamperes were used. In ten trials, the uninfected daughters were cloned from the infected parent. No appreciable difference was seen at the different current levels.

Example III

Seven samples of *ficus elastica* from a parent known to be infected were set up in nutrient agar solution at 37°C. In particular, group A consisted of three plant clones in test tubes with new silver wires, electrically stimulated as described in Example I. Group B consisted of two plant clones in test tubes set up as in Example I, but with old wires, i.e., not stimulated at this time but previously stimulated at some earlier time. Group C consisted of two plant clones in test tubes with no electrodes, and therefore served as a control group. Electrical current was supplied to Group A, according to the procedure of Example I for 92.5 hours. When the electrical current was turned off, the control group showed contamination, and both groups A and B were clear. Seven days after the electrical current was turned off, all three groups showed contamination. Thus, the presence of stimulated or formerly stimulated electrodes delayed the appearance of bacteria well beyond its appearance in the control group.

Example IV

Ficus elastica bacteria in the form of a gram negative rod of unknown type were cultured into agar onto a Petri dish provided with five silver wire anodes and a common silver wire cathode. The results are summarized in Table 1 as follows:

TABLE 1

Electrode Number	Measured Anode Current @ 25°C	Results	Anode Color
1	2.479 uA	cleared area 22mm x 10mm	black
2	0.734 uA	cleared area 15mm x 10mm	black
3	0.732 uA	cleared area	black
4	0	no cleared area	bright
5	0	no cleared area	bright

As indicated, the currents are in microamperes.

Example V

The procedure of Experiment IV was repeated using bacteria from infected raspberry plants. This was a gram negative diplo-cocci of unknown type. The results were the same as for Experiment IV. All three stimulated electrodes killed the bacteria, and the residual effect from unstimulated, used electrodes also killed the bacteria. The unstimulated, new electrodes (i.e., electrodes numbers 4 and 5), showed no cleared area, indicating no killing.

The foregoing establishes that the method and apparatus of the present invention provides a germicidal effect on plant bacteria by means of electrically stimulated silver anodes, and the foregoing also indicates that residual effects from recently stimulated electrodes also are germicidal. In both approaches, there was no apparent damage to the host plant.

A related consideration is preventing or minimizing systemic infection of the parent plant. This may be achieved by the use of microscopic samples to attempt to get through silver ion infusion into the parent cells by the use of longer term electrical stimulation to try to infuse the silver ions up into the plant capillaries, and by periodically pruning off all possible growth to excise infected material, thereby leaving only a sterile structure. Since small samples have much less probability of surviving, there may well be an optimum sample size with the best probability of survival balanced against the best probability of avoiding infection.

Another area of use of the method and apparatus of the present invention is control of nonbacterial pathogens such as tumor cells and virus infections that are not readily controlled by antibiotics or by conventional sterilizing techniques, and in a manner that does not cause death to the host plant. In particular, there is a class of viruslike pathogens called viroids which are RNA structures having no protein encasement. The viroid is only 1/100th the size of a virus, and since it is a naked RNA structure without the protein sheath that characterizes a virus, the viroid is impervious to antibodies and can withstand boiling water for about twelve minutes without damage. It also seems to be able to withstand very low temperatures. The viroid has a very long incubation period of from about six months to several years. Six plant diseases have been traced to viroids and represent a real hazard to the California citrus industry. The diseases have also been found in some New York State crops. One animal disease, scrapie in sheep, is now suspect.

The method and apparatus of the present invention as described herein was employed for the killing of a viroid pathogen as illustrated in the following example.

Example VI

Using a similar apparatus arrangement, a clone from a chrysanthemum known to be infected with a viroid (chrysanthemum stunt) was introduced into a modified Murashiga shoot media (GIBCO # 500–1124) previously introduced to the container 10, with the clone resting on the pure silver anode wire loop 20. About one microampere was passed through the silver anode during the two-week growth period of the clone. The plant grew well and developed leaves and roots. At the conclusion, the clone was pulverized, introduced into a gel, and subjected to gel electrophoresis (a process by which an electrical voltage is placed across a column; ions of different molecular weight migrate at different rates in bands, thus identifying the component). No viroid band was seen, suggesting that the silver ion environment had killed the viroid pathogen. This is a preliminary result, subject to confirmation by repetition.

The foregoing accomplishment of the electrical killing of a viroid may assume considerable clinical importance should viroids be found associated with human disease. Even for use with plant reproduction techniques, the ability of the method and apparatus of the present invention to assure a noninfected clone from a viroid infected parent is of considerable economic importance.

Another area of use of the method and apparatus of the present invention is the electrical killing of animal bacteria by anodically generated silver ions using extremely low current levels, such as those as low as 25 nanoamperes d.c. This is illustrated in the following example.

Example VII

Glass Petri dishes were prepared by drilling six to eight holes through the sides with a CO_2 laser or with a butane microtorch. A pure silver anode wire, insulated by a silicone sheath, was inserted through each hole and sealed in place with silicone cement such as Dow Corning medical adhesive "A." The wires were 0.01 inch in diameter. Two centimeters of the length of each wire extended beyond the silicone sheath. A large-area central helix of pure silver having a diameter of 0.02 inch and a length of about 10cm served as a common cathode. Each anode wire was connected through a current-limiting resistor to the positive terminal of a six volt battery. This provided a different level of current to each anode. One or two anodes were always left unconnected, i.e., zero current, as controls.

The dishes were sterilized by autoclave and then filled about 5mm deep with a sterile agar preparation. An animal bacteria culture was then introduced and allowed to grow for twenty-four hours at 37°C, producing a semiopaque cloud of bacterial colonies. With some trials new clean wires were used and the battery was connected after bacterial growth was complete. With others, the battery was connected immediately upon inoculation of the media. With still others, used dishes were cleared of media, washed, autoclaved, and refilled with new media. The current was measured with a digital microammeter in some cases and calculated in others from voltage and resistor data, making suitable allowance for some voltage polarization loss at the metal/media interface.

The results were as follows: With new wires, cleared areas (killed bacteria) developed within twenty-four hours out to 5mm from each stimulated anode. No clearing developed about the cathode, and no clearing developed about new unstimulated anodes. Residual clearing

developed about previously stimulated anodes which were rerun a second time in new media. Some clearing was observed as low as 25 nanoamperes. More clearing was developed by higher currents. Above 100 nanoamperes only modestly larger areas were cleared. At 1000 nanoamperes only about 10 percent more area was cleared that at 100 nanoamperes. When stimulation was applied immediately upon inoculation, areas within 5mm of stimulated anodes remained clear.

THE CLARENCE EXPERIMENTS

We collaborated with Becker's group and extended some of their work to lower current levels in our own laboratories. Much of this work was accomplished by biology teacher Janine Torba and her students in the biology laboratory of Clarence Central High School in 1980–81. We wish here to acknowledge the help and enthusiasm of these students in performing the experiments that led to the conclusions of this chapter. (Two of these students later went on to medical school.)

Spadero had reported germicidal effects of electrically driven silver anodes, down to 40 nA on *E. coli*.[4] We repeated and confirmed his work. Our vehicle was a number of 6-inch Petri pyrex glass dishes in whose walls we drilled holes with a CO_2 laser. Silver wires were passed through the holes and sealed with silicone medical adhesive. One wire was spiraled in the center as a cathode and six were spaced at equal intervals radially around the cathode and adjacent to the dish wall. A physiological saline agar solution was prepared, inoculated with *E. coli,* and grown to turbidity about the immersed wires.

Anodic currents of different levels were passed through the wires. Current level was maintained by the use of ±1 percent precision resistors in series with a 6v battery. Tests showed that, at the miniscule current levels that were used, the voltage drop across the incubation cell was an insignificant fraction of the battery voltage. Thus, the current was closely approximated by:

$$I = \frac{6V}{R}$$

The germicidal effect was detected by the clearing of an elliptical area around the anode electrode. This work is further detailed under Example VII.

Becker et al.[5] and Spadero et al.[6] had done considerable work using this principle with a number of electrode metals on a number of pathogens. We think it significant that silver, of all the metals tested, was the only one to produce a consistent germicidal effect at nanoampere/microampere current levels, and then only through anode electrodes.

We gave considerable thought as to why no clearing was seen more than $\frac{1}{2}$ cm away from an anode wire, even at 1000nA. We decided to try to determine a) whether the germicidal effect was the electrical current "electrocuting" the bacteria or, b) if the sole function of the electrical current was that of corroding the wire to create silver ions, which then chemically killed the bacteria; in other words, was the germicidal effect electrical or chemical?

We decided to move the cathode very close to the anode and observe any change in the shape of the cleared area. The electrical field would then be markedly disturbed, and the zero potential line would fall halfway between the closely-spaced anode and cathode. If the germicidal effect were electrical, this would distort the pattern of the cleared area from the previously seen elliptical shape. If the germicidal action were purely chemical, the cleared area would not change in shape. The results showed a cleared area very little changed from before. In fact the cathode actually lay well within the cleared area. Thus we concluded that the ger-

---

THE WAY IT WAS

Word got around the school of what we were doing. The other science teachers started dropping in with advice and observations. Then the principal dropped in. All this intensified the students' interest. I got pretty excited about it myself. Each day I'd rush over to the school to see what grew the night before. One of the kids, a problem student, wound up in my own shop after school, building the electronics.

*   *   *

During a discussion of a proposed WGLtd. research budget, I was doing a little (instructional) bragging to #1 son Warren (later the president of WGLtd.) about how much work we got done on this project for so little money. He replied, "Sure, because you used the school district's facilities for the biology and my $70,000 laser to drill the holes."

Some people are just too realistic!

micidal action was purely chemical and the only function of the electrical current was to generate silver ions. The bacteria didn't seem to know that the electric field was there.

With the meager facilities available to us and our own limited knowledge of bioelectrochemistry, I thought these experiments represented a commendable piece of work for a high school science class. It was a good experience (and not even on a federal grant).

KILLING OF PLANT BACTERIA: THE GRAND ISLAND EXPERIMENTS

Using the same Petri dishes, the anode wires were shortened and curved into small 2mm circles. A 1mm tissue clone of *ficus elastica* known to be infected with a rod bacteria was placed on the anode loop in the agar. All previous attempts to disinfect the clone by standard means had failed. One microampere of DC current was applied for two hours. The clone was then retrieved and placed into a fresh test tube containing standard tissue culture medium. Three successive generations of genetically identical daughters were then propagated from this clone. All proved to be disease-free. Further details of this work are spelled out in Examples I–V. The experiments were performed at the Grand Island Biological Co. by Dr. Don Tartock and David Tricoli.

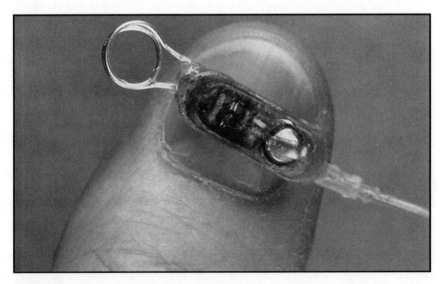

Infection control device for implant in mice.

Subsequently, we built a packaged stimulator which could be put into a test tube along with tissue culture medium. The battery for the stimulator was a new 3.0v, 30mahr lithium silver vanadium pentoxide cell which can operate successfully at autoclave temperatures. The circuit was a simple but effective FET current regulator which could hold at 1uA ±1 percent with load variations from zero ohms to over one megohm. We have autoclaved some of these stimulators over fifty times without adverse effects.

A current of 1uA is probably more than is needed. We have seen adequate killing of plant bacteria at 0.2uA (along with improved plant growth) but have seen some plants killed at 2uA. Such a stimulator is reusable hundreds of times. It is our practice to read the open-circuit voltage (OCV) on a high-impedance voltmeter (over 10 megohms input resistance) after each autoclave, and to record current from a digital nanoammeter.

KILLING AND/OR INHIBITING OF TUMOR CELLS: THE SYRACUSE EXPERIMENTS

J. Spadero et al. reported the killing of leukemia-like ascites, floating tumor cells from mice, in vitro, with electrically produced Ag^+ ions.[7] He additionally found the following[8]:

1.) Ascites cells, electrically treated with Ag^+ ions in vitro, showed the following viabilities with tripan iodine uptake indicators:

current	duration	viability
0.25 ua	5 hours	95%
1.0	5	35%
2.5	2	93%
2.5	4	0%
2.0	3	33%
2.0	4	0%

It is notable that three to four hours of stimulation were necessary to get any positive results.

2.) The above experiment was repeated in Dr. Spadero's laboratory, but with a bioassay (to determine its effectiveness on organisms), by injecting the treated cells into healthy Swiss Webster mice.

current	duration	viability
0 ua	0 hours	all died by day 28
0.2	4	4 of 10 survived 46 days
2.0	4	all survived to 53 days
20.0	4	all survived to 53 days

It would appear that in vitro treatment of ascites cells with anodically generated silver ions renders them incapable of infecting mice.

3.) To continue this work in vivo, six Swiss Webster mice were inoculated with a strain of Erlich's ascites tumor cells of original human origin which were originally obtained from Dr. Erlich at the Roswell Park Memorial Cancer Institute in Buffalo, New York. Three of these mice also received small subcutaneously implantable electronic stimulators. These stimulators were similar to the plant stimulators previously described but were much smaller and delivered 10ua. The battery was a zinc silver mercury watch battery with a calculated life of 3,000 hours. Both anode and cathode were 0.010"D pure silver wire loops of two turns each, ¼" D. Results from these tests were inconclusive and not repeatable, some suggesting a definite regression of the tumors and others not.

IMPLANTED DEVICES AT SYRACUSE, NEW YORK

In collaboration with Robert Becker and Joseph Spadero, we built dozens of miniature implantable devices. Most used zinc mercury hearing aid batteries, but some used lithium silver vanadium pentoxide cells. Two of the latter stimulators were autoclaved fifty times without apparent damage.

We used a constant-current regulator circuit, using a field effect transistor (FET; a special type of transistor with a very high input impedance). Very few FETs operate at a gate voltage of 0.5v, which is necessary if the total power supply is only 1.5v. However, we found one that worked very well. The circuit and performance are shown on the following page for a 100nA configuration.

A number of these devices were made and implanted in mice. Most were used in a program in extension of previous work by Spadero et al.,[9] which suggested that silver ion deposition could considerably extend the lifetime of mice in which ascites tumors had been implanted. A first trial confirmed this earlier work, but subsequent trials were inconclusive. The Syracuse Veterans Administration Hospital orthopedic research laboratory was closed after the retirement of Dr. Becker, its director, and no further efforts with our devices were undertaken.

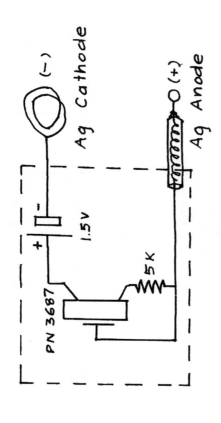

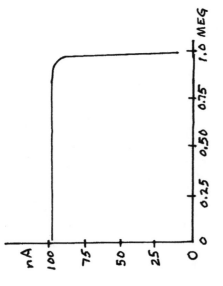

Circuit for a 100nA configuration.

THE SUNYAB EXPERIMENTS

A similar program was undertaken in the Biophysics Department of the State University of New York at Buffalo in collaboration with Dr. Michael Anbar, director, and Dr. Rath. This involved regression of chondrosarcoma tumors in rats. Again, one test suggested an affirmative result, but following tests did not reinforce the earlier findings. A change of personnel left no one in the department doing this kind of work, and we did not continue it.

Each of these projects was carried along until it became clear that there was to be no clear cut, "quick fix." Each of these projects would make interesting thesis work, and perhaps this chapter will encourage someone to continue our efforts. However, the effort involved is beyond our own facilities. Since, at the moment, our primary interests lie in other directions, we are not continuing with it.

VIROID EXPERIMENTS AT CORNELL UNIVERSITY

Several devices were built for Dr. Kenneth Horst of the Department of Plant Pathology of Cornell University for experiments in inhibiting the growth of viroids. In plants, they are responsible for a number of potato, tomato, chrysanthemum, and citrus diseases. In animals, a viroidlike disease, scrapie, is a uniformly fatal central nervous system (CNS) disease of sheep. There also exist a number of "slow virus" diseases in humans for which the pathogen has never been visualized. They are characterized by long incubation times (up to twenty years), CNS degradation, and a fatal prognosis. The most spectacular of these is kuru, a disease found

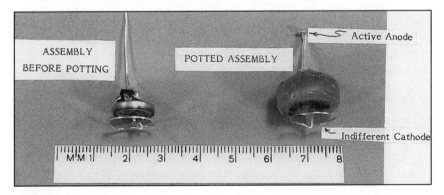

Sterilization module for test tube.

among New Guinea cannibals. The disease was passed from one generation to the next by a funeral ceremony in which the widow had to eat the
brain of the deceased. There have been no new kuru cases in over twenty
years since the practice of cannibalism was discouraged. (Later work has
attributed to *prions* what we thought might be attributed to viroids.)

B. Sigurdsson first described "slow diseases" in sheep in Iceland.[10]
The sheep were first introduced in the 1930s as a single lot of Karakul
sheep from a farm in Halle, Germany. Icelandic sheep had been introduced from Scandinavia a thousand years before and had been completely isolated for all that time. They had acquired no immunity to
many diseases, and by 1940 the situation was so bad that it was necessary to slaughter all of the Icelandic sheep to eliminate the diseases. Sigurdsson suggests as criteria for slow disease: 1) a very long incubation
period of latency; 2) a regular protracted course of the disease, ending in
death; and 3) limitation of the infection to a single host species.

The slow virus diseases are also known as "subacute spongiform
encephalopathies." Many investigators have noted the similarity of
a number of diseases to that of the Icelandic sheep. Kimberlin lists
the following[11]:

Scrapie in sheep
Visna in sheep
Maedi in sheep
Kuru in humans
Creutzfeld-Jakob disease in humans
Transmissible Mink Encephalopathy (TME)
Progressive multifocal leucoencephalopathy (PML) in humans
Subacute sclerosing panencephalitis in humans
Multiple sclerosis in humans

Pollard adds to this list familial Alzheimer's disease and progressive
nuclear palsy.[12] In addition, J. Henson in Kenya suggests some other
human diseases in which slow viruses have been proven or suggested to
be etiologic agents[13]:

In humans:
     SLE
     Polyarteritis nodoso
     Rheumatoid arthritis
     Viral hepatitis
and in animals:
     Equine infectious anemia
     Hog cholera
     African swine fever
     Lymphocytic choriomeningitis

It is interesting to note that African swine fever has been implicated in the high prevalence of AIDS among Haitians. Fucillo adds some "chronic degenerative diseases of unknown etiology": multiple sclerosis; amyotrophic lateral sclerosis; Parkinson's disease; and presenile dementia.[14]

Thus, it is apparent that the slow virus diseases are quite widespread, but much has been learned about slow viruses in the twenty-five years since this was written, and readers should not be misled into accepting the above material. Kimberlin states that the scrapie agent is very resistant to heat, nuclear radiation, and ultraviolet radiation.[15] A brain preparation has been known to survive 100°C for thirty minutes without losing its infectivity. Gibbs states that kuru and Creutzfeldt-Jakob agents are not affected by 20×10^6 rads of Co^{60} radiation and are resistant to storage in 10 percent formaldehyde.[16] He stated in discussion that a paraffin imbedded sample of transmissible mink encephalopathy had resided in a desk drawer for over six years, and another sample had resided in 10 percent formaldehyde for over three years without losing infectivity.[17] A Zurich surgical group had studied Creutzfeldt-Jakob disease in human brains clinically with gold electrodes, washing them between procedures in alcohol. At least two subsequent disease-free patients contracted the disease and died. A full autoclave procedure will kill the agents, however.

We thought our infection control devices might have some application here if we could demonstrate a favorable effect on inhibition of chrysanthemum stunt, a viroid disease. Again, some suggestions of effect were seen initially, but the results were inconclusive. Present efforts in this direction have moved over into an investigation into mycoplasmic pathogens. This work is further detailed in Example VI.

Silver Toxicity

Silver, being a heavy metal, naturally raises some concern about toxicity in the body. Fortunately, we find no evidence in the literature for concern over the miniscule quantities used for infection control devices. However, ingestion of larger quantities can produce some cosmetic effects. Agyria is a condition in which persons exposed to or ingesting significant quantities of silver can develop a grey-blue cast to their skin, particularly on skin areas which are exposed to direct sunlight. This condition was first noted in England where silver was used in manufacturing "crackers."

British workers in the cracker factories who were exposed to silver salts for years absorbed silver into their systems and developed the cosmetic discoloring of their skin typical of agyria. It is a chronic condition that was of major concern to the British industrial medical community.

THE WAY IT WAS

An American "cracker" is an English "biscuit." A British "cracker" is a twist of paper with pull-tabs on the ends, and it contains a small explosive charge. When the tabs are pulled, a very gratifying "bang" results. British children look forward to getting them in their stockings at Christmas time.

J. Harker et al. reported a study of sixteen cases of occupational agyria.[18] Some were from contact with silver in the production of silver nitrate. One other case was a girl who made "crackers" with silver fulminate and wet her fingers with her mouth to facilitate handling the parts. Only one of the sixteen cases investigated had ever sought medical assistance and all eventually died of unrelated conditions. Harker states that the processes which led to manual contact with the silver had been made obsolete by 1935.

H. Prose reported an electron microscopic study of human agyria from samples taken from a patient who had taken excessive amounts of nasal argerol.[19] Prose also makes reference to the "Blue Man" of the Barnum and Bailey circus who represented a case of agyria. Prose found silver combined with sulfur in basement membranes surrounding sweat glands, and in the kidneys. Only rarely was silver found elsewhere. He found no pathology related to silver.

L. Rich et al. reported a patient referred for cyanotic heart disease.[20] He was a sixty-nine-year-old Caucasian who had been taking Neo-Silvol nose drops (which are 20 percent silver iodide) six times daily for sinusitis. He was subsequently correctly diagnosed as having agyria, with no immediate heart problem. Rich mentions that agyria is not directly due to silver, but rather is the result of an increased production of melanin in the skin, triggered by the presence of excessive silver.

The sole literature reference we can find on detrimental effects of silver is R. Cooper who reports adverse effects of silver electrodes in the brain.[21] This, however, is not a systemic problem nor has it been reported by others. There exists an extensive history of silver pacemaker electrodes, used both by General Electric four decades ago and more recently by Medtronic, Inc., with no reported adverse effects.

Silver salts are no longer used in "crackers." Other silver workers are generally protected from direct contact with their work, and agyria is rarely seen today. It is fortunate that we have significant long-term data

THE WAY IT WAS

About four decades ago we were seeking nonpolarizable ECG skin electrodes for our astronaut instrumentation. Ordinary metallic ECG electrodes generate up to 300 mv of interface voltage which is heavily modulated by electrode motion. This can swamp out the 1 mv R wave you are seeking. The best we could find were the Beckman silver, silver-chloride electrodes of C. Luchina.[22] We made them by mixing together equal quantities of powdered silver and powdered silver chloride, inserting a silver wire, and then pressing the mix into a 5mm D x 2mm pellet at 20 tons pressure. Our press was a frame of structural steel, made by Richard Hagele, with a movable bar depressed by a 20 ton hydraulic truck jack, operated by hand. This worked fine and we made thousands of the electrodes at MG Electronics Inc. for hospital coronary care units. They worked on a principle of having a common ion across each chemical interface. This gave a chloride ion exchange across the skin barrier (best results were obtained with a needle prick under the electrode), a common chloride ion from the skin surface into the silver chloride, and a common silver ion from the silver chloride into the silver wire. The silver, being a metallic system, could generate no additional interface voltages. Such electrodes, face-to-face, would show less than 1 mv of DC offset potential after an overnight soak in saline. When properly applied, they could be struck with the flat of the hand without generating more than a millivolt of artifact.

We thought that if silver were that good, gold or platinum should be better, so we made some gold, gold-chloride and some platinum, platinum-chloride electrodes. They worked fine for a couple of hours but then polarized heavily. Microscopic examination revealed that all the chloride had dissolved out of the pellet, leaving a pure metal spongy matrix.[23]

to reassure us that silver toxicity is not a problem, even at documented exposures that are orders of magnitude greater than could be experienced with infection control devices.

We have presented a number of isolated literature references and experiences of our own in infection control by electrically generated silver ions. This mode of infection control is rarely used today, but we think that some aspects of it may be worth further investigation. It is a fascinating interplay of chemistry, physics, engineering, and pharmacology. We hope that perhaps something we have said may generate interest on someone's part.

We are indebted to Dr. Peter Lord for pointing us towards the agyria references, and to Mrs. Jean Wilds, the British wife of one of our vice presidents, for explanations of "crackers."

Gold Ion Treatment

One of the treatments for rheumatoid arthritis involves intramuscular injection of gold salts. Over a period of a year or so, an attempt is made to build the systemic level of gold up to about one gram. This treatment is often ineffective and is sometimes accompanied by severe side effects. Very little is known about the mechanism of beneficial effects when they do occur. It is not known whether it is the high systemic level of gold that benefits the patient or if it is the fraction of the total load that comes to rest in the affected joint. Should the latter be the case, it would appear preferable to administer a much smaller total dose of gold directly in the affected joint. This might achieve the desired effect without the severe side effects that can accompany higher doses. We thought about using a small implantable ion generator, much like those we had used in silver ion infection control and in osteogenesis. Faraday's Law states that for each ion of gold generated, one, two, or five electrons will be consumed from the battery, depending on the valence of the particular gold involved in the reaction. The gold, in ionic form, should remain in the tissue in much higher concentration than in the case of silver, since the gold salts that are used are so much more soluble (ionizable) than silver chloride.

Gold is usually combined in a monovalent form with sulfur, as aurothioglucose, or gold sodium thiomalate, both of which are about 50 percent gold. These substances are given by intramuscular injection, although an oral version, auranofin, is used in Europe. Adverse toxic side effects are seen in 25 percent to 50 percent of patients treated, with about 0.4 percent mortality due to the gold treatment (chrysotherapy). It is interesting that a grey to blue skin pigmentation is sometimes seen, particularly in skin areas that are exposed to sunlight. This is similar to the agyria seen from extended contact with silver salts, although no silver is involved here. About 60 percent to 70 percent of patients see improvement in symptoms, 15 percent show no response, and about 15 percent to 20 percent experience toxic reactions which require reduction or cessation of medication.[24]

J. Flower et al. states that gold is entrained in part in phagosomes in the synovial membrane.[25] R. Gerber et al. mention that during treatment the concentration of gold in the synovial fluid (joint lubricant) is about half that in plasma.[26] If indeed the gold acts in the inflamed joint, then our implantable ion generator may well add another treatment for the rheumatologist, one that avoids toxic side effects by depositing the gold only where it is needed. Local application of such treatment might find use in athletic medicine in connection with atheroscopy to reduce inflammation of injured cartilage.

We convinced ourselves that the implantable gold ion generator was buildable and would be safe and effective. The further questions in physiological safety and efficacy and best mode of application would require extensive animal and clinical investigation. Since we found no one interested in such an effort, we wrote all our ideas up into a patent application and put it on the shelf for awhile.[27]

Silver-Nylon Cloth

Dr. Dwight Harken, an eminent Boston surgeon, recalls Dr. Cushman using silver foil as a bactericidal wound dressing about six decades ago. Some investigators have considered weaving silver wires into nylon cloth, or using nylon thread which is silver coated in weaving the cloth. Such cloth can be used as a wound dressing and electrically stimulated to produce a germicidal silver ion deposition. Cloth of this type is made by Ritter Fauber (Sybron) of Rochester, New York, and has been the subject of investigation by J. Spadero and R. Becker,[28] A. Marino,[29] and L. Deitch.[30] This appears to be an attractive concept, but we have had no experience with it.

In summary, we are excited about our in vitro experimental work but we are not encouraged by our in vivo results. There seems to be some indication that silver ion deposition is beneficial in infection control, in tumor regression, and in viroid control. It is also certain that the treatment is far from 100 percent effective and that the reasons for this are unknown. None of the work described here was funded by grants and most of the time spent by participants was volunteered. A more massive, better funded effort might have solved some of the problems.

NOTES

1. K. Horst et al., *Plant Disease* 64 (1980): 186.
2. W. Greatbatch, "Method and Apparatus for Electronic Control of Infection." U.S. Patent 4,291,125, 1981.

3. Ibid.

4. J. Spadero and R. Becker, "Some Specific Cellular Effects of Electrically Injected Silver and Gold Ions." *Bioelectrochem. and Bioenergetics* 3 (1976): 49.

5. R. Becker and J. Spadero, "Treatment of Orthopedic Infections with Electrically Generated Silver Ions." *J. Bone and Joint Surgery* 60-A, no. 7 (1978): 871.

6. J. Spadero, T. Berger, S. Barranco, S. Chapin, and R. Becker, "Antibacterial Effects of Silver Electrodes with Weak Electric Current." *Antibacterial Agents and Chemotherapy* (1974): 637.

7. Ibid.

8. J. Spadero, Personal communication, 1978.

9. J. Spadero et al., "Antibacterial Effects of Silver Electrodes with Weak Electric Current," 637.

10. B. Sigurdsson, *British Vet. J.* 110 (1954): 341.

11. R. Kimberlin, *Slow Virus Diseases of Animals and Man* 1, no. 4 (Amsterdam: North-Holland Elsevier, 1976), 6.

12. M. Pollard, *Perspectives in Virology* 11, edited by M. Pollard (New York: Raven Press, 1978).

13. J. Henson, J. Gorham, T. McGuire, and T. Crawford, "Pathology and Pathogenesis of Aleutian Disease." In *Slow Virus Diseases of Animals and Man 9*, edited by R. H. Kimberlin(Amsterdam: North-Holland Elsevier, 1976), 202.

14. D. Fucillo, J. Kurent, and J. Sever, "Slow Virus Diseases." *Ann. Review of Microbiology* 28 (1974): 231.

15. Kimberlin, *Slow Virus Diseases of Animals and Man,* 6.

16. C. Gibbs and D. Gadjusek, "Atypical Viruses as the Cause of Sporadic Epidemic and Familial Chronic Disease in Man: Slow Viruses and Human Disease." *Perspectives in Virology* 11, edited by M. Pollard (New York: Raven Press, 1978), 161.

17. Ibid.

18. J. Harker and D. Hunter, "Occupational Agyria." *British J. Dermatology and Syphilis* (1935): 441.

19. H. Prose, "An Electron Microscope Study of Human Agyria." *Am. J. Pathology* 42 (1963): 293.

20. L. Rich, W. Epinette, and W. Nasser, "Agyria Presenting as Cyanotic Heart Disease." *Am. J. Cardiol.* 30 (1972): 290.

21. R. Cooper and H. Crow, "Toxic Effect on Intra-cerebral Electrodes." *Medical and Biol. Engin.* 4 (1966): 575.

22. C. Luchina, "A Vectorcardiographic Lead System and Physiological Electrode System for Dynamic Readout." *Aerospace Medicine* 33, no. 6 (1962): 722. See also U.S. Patents 3,137,291 and 3,170,459.

23. W. Greatbatch, "Gold, Gold Chloride and Platinum, Platinum Chloride Compressed Pellet Physiological Electrodes." *Proc. 17th Annual Conference of Engineering in Medicine and Biology* (IEEE), Cleveland, 1964.

24. J. Flower, S. Moncada, and J. Vane, "Analgesic Antipyretics and Anti-inflammatory Agents." In *The Pharmacological Basis of Therapeutics* 5 (New York: Macmillan, 1980), 713–17.

25. Ibid.

26. R. Gerber, H. Paulus, R. Bluestone, and M. Lederer, "Kinetics of Aurothiomalate in Serum and Synovial Fluid." *Arthrit. Rheum.* 15 (1972): 625.

27. W. Greatbatch, "Method and Apparatus for Direct Injection of Gold Ions Into Tissue Such as Bone." U.S. Patent 4,405,311, 1983.

28. J. Spadero et al., "Some Specific Cellular Effects of Electrically Injected Silver and Gold Ions."

29. A. Marino, V. Malaknok, E. Deitch, and J. Albright, "Electrical Properties of Silver-nylon." *Trans 3rd Annual Meeting BRAGS*, San Francisco III (1983): 36.

30. E. Deitch, A. Marino, V. Malaknok, and J. Albright, "Electrical Augmentation of the Antibacterial Activity of Silver-nylon." *Trans. 3rd Annual Meeting BRAGS*, San Francisco, III (1983): 59.

31. J. Spadero and R. Becker, "Some Specific Cellular Effects of Electrically Injected Silver and Gold Ions," 49.

32. J. Cowlishaw, J. Spadero, and R. Becker, "Inhibition of Enzyme Induction in *E. Coli* by Anodic Silver." *J. Bioelectricity* 1, no. 3 (1982): 295.

FOR FURTHER READING

Ellis, F., and S. Andrews, "Method of In-vivo Sterilization of Surgical Implantables." U.S. Patent 4,027,393, 1977.

Gage, A., Personal communication, 1983.

Spadero, J., D. Webster, and S. Chase, "Direct Current Activation of Bacteriostatic Silver Electrodes." *Trans. 3rd Annual Meeting BRAGS*, San Francisco, III (1983): 37.

ADDENDUM

After completing this chapter in 1983, we submitted it to good friend Joe Spadero at the Upstate Medical Center in Syracuse, New York, for peer review.

Dr. Spadero called to my attention two papers I had completely missed: Spadero et al. (1976) extended some of their previous work on silver ion generation down to 40nA and found that bacterial action is present, but at a decreasing degree, under 100nA. Spadero attributes the action to interference with membrane-related activity. He also studied the effect of anodically generated silver ions on the induction of beta-galactosidase in *E. coli* growing in a glycerol-salts minimum medium. He shows that production of the enzyme was inhibited almost completely at the anode within twenty minutes of beginning the treatment, but unaffected at the cathode. This effect seems to be a precursor of the bacteriostatic effect of silver and occurs at ionic concentrations of silver known to be much lower than that of marginally lethal silver salts. Thus, he infers the membrane-related activity. This work is further detailed by Cowlishaw et al. (1982).

Spadero et al. (1976) also described the anti-inflammatory effect of about 10^{-7} moles of gold ions, anodically generated in arthritic rabbit knees by a voltage of + 0.9v applied for two hours to gold wires implanted in the joints. Qualitative postmortem evaluation demonstrated reduced invasion of cartilage, reduced synovial hypertrophy, and clarity of synovial fluid.

10

IMPLANTABLE DRUG INFUSION PUMPS

INTRODUCTION

In the recent past, new terms have entered the medico-pharmaceutical literature, terms such as genetic engineering and drug infusion delivery systems. Instrumentation and engineering are playing an increasing role in their development. The result is a literal revolution in the manufacture and delivery of pharmaceuticals to the patient. Drug infusion devices are being used for administration of heparin anticoagulant; administration of cancer therapy drugs; programmed administration of insulin; and administration of antiarrythmia cardiac drugs.

ENGINEERING IN DRUG MANUFACTURING

Most drugs were originally derived from natural sources. The quality control in their manufacture was subject to batch-to-batch variations and to economic conditions of supply and demand. It is also necessary to consider possible political instability in the source countries. Costs, quality, and consistency are usually much improved when the drug can be synthesized from chemicals. Economies of scale then become easier to achieve, and the physician is assured of a more consistent end effect. Side effects from trace impurities which may unexpectedly appear in the natural raw product are more likely to be better controlled or even eliminated by synthetic production.

The term "genetic engineering" is not truly nuts-and-bolts engineering, as engineers have understood it, but it still implies an engineering of the genetic structure to obtain new properties as well as unknown products.

On January 11, 1922, a fourteen-year-old boy, Leonard Thomson, was the first diabetes patient to receive a new hormone, insulin, developed by Frederick Banting in Toronto, Canada. Within two years the University of Toronto and the Eli Lilly Company were filling the needs of 10,000 diabetics. By 1936, the Hagedorn company in Copenhagen had succeeded in modifying the basic insulin to provide slow acting insulin. By 1981, Lilly was providing no less than fourteen different insulin products, all made from the pancreas glands of cattle or swine.

It is estimated that in 1981 there were sixty million diabetics in the world. Of twenty-five million of these in developed countries, ten million remained undiagnosed. Less than ten percent of the world's diabetics are under insulin treatment. But diabetic patients who normally would have died in their teens without treatment are now living more normal lifetimes and having children, many of whom unfortunately show genetic tendencies towards the disease. Thus the number of diabetics in the United States is growing at twice the rate of the normal population. There is concern on the part of some that the natural sources will prove inadequate to supply the demand for insulin, although a National Institutes of Health (NIH) report (NIH-78-1588, 1978) stated that no shortage is foreseen over the next two decades.

Events that led to new hope for a virtually limitless supply of insulin began in 1953 when James Watson and Francis Crick announced their Nobel Prize winning discovery of the double helix structure of DNA. In rapid succession thereafter it was shown that 1) a bacterium, *Escherichia coli*, used DNA as a template to replicate itself; 2) the DNA molecules could be cut from two different organisms and recombined; 3) a rat insulin gene could be spliced into DNA; and 4) in 1978 the Genentec and Eli Lilly companies announced that they had created synthetic genes and inserted them into *E. coli* to produce human insulin. Clinical trials began two years later and by March 1982, nine hundred patients had been treated with human insulin (recombinant DNA, or rDNA) therapy. FDA approval followed in late 1982.

Recombinant DNA production* is a fermentation process in which engineering design and engineering instrumentation play a strong part. Although in recent years many technical changes have occurred in this age-old process, the principles for fermentation of recombinant DNA organisms remain essentially the same as those used for antibiotics since the 1950s. The basic equipment consists of closed stainless steel vessels

---

*The process described here is largely 1980s technology.

fitted with agitators to mix the contents and aid in aeration. Compressed air that has been filtered to remove contaminating organisms is pumped into the fermenter to provide necessary oxygen for growth. Metabolic heat is removed by a cooling jacket.

Instrumentation and monitoring of the operating system are carried out continually and include microbiological sampling of the exhaust systems after filtration, sampling of the operator environment, and frequent integrity testing of the filtration systems. Modern instrumentation monitors variables such as fermenter temperature, air flow, pressure, pH, dissolved oxygen, feed rates of various nutrients, and composition of exhaust gases.

Antibiotic fermenters were originally designed primarily to protect the fermentation from contaminating organisms. To adapt them to fermentations with recombinant organisms, they are modified to contain the fermentation organism more completely by filtration, incineration of the exhaust gases, containment of the agitator seal, sampling and inoculating with a closed system, and chemical or thermal sterilization of the fermenter contents before processing. The protocols for operating fermentation vessels with microorganisms containing recombinant DNA are somewhat more complex because of the containment features for inoculation, sampling, and so on.

A particular strain, *E. coli* K12 is safe, nonpathogenic, and cannot support itself outside the laboratory environment. In the future, one may expect that other host organisms such as streptomyces or saccharomyces will be used industrially. Again, the criterion of inability of the laboratory-modified strains to survive in their natural habitat must be met.

Most insulin used in 1983 was a mixture of naturally derived porcine and bovine insulin. Biosynthetic human insulin (BHI), developed by Genentec and licensed to Eli Lilly for production, was the first example of a clinically useful product of recombinant DNA technology. J. Skyler et al. have extensively surveyed the literature, studying the equivalence of BHI to purified porcine insulin.[1] He concludes that they are essentially clinically equivalent. He suggests that BHI may be superior in terms of immunogenicity (the effect of genetics on immunity) because of its synthetic source and that because of this, it will nearly certainly be superior to bovine insulin. Also, the availability of BHI removes the possibility of potential shortages of insulin. The creation of BHI was a feat important in its own right as a major scientific advance and foretold the successful development and application of untold numbers of other synthetic drugs in the near future.

There is a growing recognition of the necessity to engineer any drug to match the requirement of the associated drug diffusion device. Three aspects stand out: 1) the chemical stability of the drug; 2) the mechanical stability of the drug; and 3) the corrosion properties of the drug. Many drugs have only a short shelf-life and must be kept under refrigeration until they are used. Some of these degrade rapidly in the warm environment of the body. To be suitable in a drug administration system, such drugs should be chemically stable for weeks and preferably for months. If one must replenish the reservoir every day with fresh material, much of the advantage over conventional subcutaneous needle injection may be lost, although some feel that the programmability of the pump will represent an improvement in patient care, even if daily refilling is required.

Many of the early insulin pumps were faulty because the insulin collected in the catheter or around the exit port. Some investigators suggested additives to counteract this. J. Bringer et al. suggested dicarboxylic amino acid additives.[2] A. Albisser et al. suggested 1.5 percent autologus serum as an additive.[3] D. Schade et al. suggested use of a polyethylene catheter and additives of polyethylene glycol or lysine to prevent coagulation.[4] None of these seem to present a satisfactory long-term solution, and more work needs to be done.*

Some investigators found the delivery of lidocaine for alleviation of heart arrythmias to be limited by viscosity as well as by the corrosive effect of the drug on the stainless steel pump. Also, several of the insulin compounds are known to be corrosive to some pump mechanisms. NOVO Industri A/S of Copenhagen has produced a monocomponent insulin which should help, in this respect.

We regard the engineering of the drug to adapt it to the drug administration device as a major and necessary part of the development of the device itself. We also believe that this drug development program is not as far advanced as much of the literature would have us believe.

The costs associated with developing a new drug and obtaining approval from the regulatory agencies for its use are escalating. M. C. Behrens of Sutro & Co. who watches Genentech, stated in the *Wall Street Journal* (August 26, 1982, 15) that the cost of getting acceptance of a new drug is now between seventeen and forty million dollars for each product.

OPEN-LOOP VERSUS CLOSED-LOOP SYSTEMS

Obviously the most desirable drug administration device would sense the need for the drug and then deliver it in exactly the dosage needed at

---

*Even by 1990 an unmodified insulin-suitable implantable insulin pump did not exist, but implantable drug pumps were commercially available for heparin and chemotherapy drugs.

precisely the correct time. Unfortunately, few sensors exist which can reliably give accurate indications of such need over extended periods of time. This is particularly true for sugar sensors.

A new class of sensors uses solid-state ion selective membranes that can pass certain ions which then approach the gate of a field effect transistor (a particular transistor design with very high input impedance). The resulting electrical charge varies the conduction of the transistor, permitting an electrical readout. Not only can such sensors measure elemental ions, but there is some indication that certain ionic molecules can also be sensed. The critical factor is the development of new membranes with the desired selective factor. To date, however, we know of no sugar sensor that can survive in the body more than a few days. Until such a sensor is developed, true closed-loop operation (sensing hyperglycemia and delivering insulin precisely as needed) of an implanted insulin pump will not be feasible.

Some investigators have, in a sense, closed this loop by frequent and periodic withdrawal and analysis of blood samples. S. Bessman et al.[5] and H. Broekhuyse et al.[6] have described such systems and termed them "closed loop." Such systems involve a five to fifteen minute delay between withdrawal and analysis of the blood sample and administration of the desired drug. We tend to question the closed-loop terminology in such a case, since the time delay between sensing and correcting the deficit puts an objectionable delay in the loop.

Alternatives to actually tightly closing the loop can involve either allowing complete patient control of the system or building a program into the device. Such a program can involve an electronic digital clock which programs the delivery of the drug according to some predetermined regimen of need. In the case of diabetes, this involves a slow, steady basal rate of insulin delivery with additional periodic programmed delivery of a single, large dose of insulin preceding a meal, the size and rate of which the patient can determine. More sophisticated programming systems involve many choices of basal rate and of bolus dosage. The present availability of the complete computer capability of a conventional desktop computer on a single, thumb-nail size, monolithic semiconductor chip permits a nearly unlimited electronic control of such a device. Also, suitable implantable power sources are readily available to run it. These factors are clearly apparent in the proliferation of highly programmable implantable drug administration devices, come of which are already well into clinical trials.

We have had a special interest in Parkinson's disease, primarily because we see a more promising opportunity to close the loop between sensing tremor or spacity and delivering corrective drug therapy. Parkinson's disease is an irreversible brain disorder that results in muscle tremor. Its fatal prognosis is inevitable, but programmed delivery of lev-udopa (a medicine to control tremors) can alleviate its uncomfortable and embarrassing tremors. Oral medication usually has a half hour delay before becoming effective, and the average patient receives perhaps three hours of relief. However, some patients receive only one half hour of relief after a half hour delay. An accidental overdose can replace the tremors with uncontrolled limb and head motions. Such patients are essentially out of control.

An interesting aspect of this disease is that the detectable error signal is electrical rather then chemical. A pair of electrodes on an appropriate muscle could detect the tremor as an AC myopotential with electrical characteristics that should permit a rather easy discrimination from the overdose myopotential signal twitches or from outside noise interference. It may well be that, because of the opportunity to sense an electrical rather than a chemical error signal, this disease, or one similar to it, may be the first to come under control with an implantable drug pump.*

ENGINEERING OF DRUG DELIVERY SYSTEMS

In the past the physician has administered drugs either in oral doses by leave in injection, or by continuous infusion through intravenous tubes. Some ambulatory patients are not adequately managed by infrequent, periodic doses and yet should not have their lifestyle restricted by bed-side intravenous infusion. Consequently, a number of portable drug infusion devices have been introduced. The earliest ones delivered a fac-tory-set, constant rate of flow. The dosage could be varied only by diluting the drug.

Administration of the drug can be by intravenous, subcutaneous, intramuscular, or intraperitoneal means. Each has its advantages and disadvantages. Intravenous means give the quickest response, but are most subject to aggregation problems with some drugs. Intraperitoneal means are attractive, particularly for drug-related cancer treatment of the liver, since this location provides a direct link to the portal system.

External Pump Design

Portable drug infusion systems are obviously external to the body, but are easily carried, usually on the patient. Many mechanical pump struc-tures have been used, ranging from motor-driven leadscrew syringes to peristaltic roller pumps, to positive displacement piston pumps, and dual

---

*However, this technology, suggested in 1983, has still not been achieved in 2000.

chamber pumps with the drug on one side of a diaphragm and a two-phase, liquid/gas fluorocarbon on the other side. The fluorocarbon evaporates as pressure drops, maintaining a relatively constant pressure on the drug chamber.

The first insulin infusion pump was the British Mill Hill Infusor. The rate of drug delivery was factory-set at two pulses per second in some models or four pulses per second in others. The piston of a motor-driven syringe was driven forward by a leadscrew. The device used a disposable syringe.

Siemans AG (of Erlangen, Germany) has introduced a portable device that uses a peristaltic pump. Probably the most used American device is by Autosyringe of Hooksett, New Hampshire. It uses a syringe pump with a variable basal rate.

Other newer models feature more sophisticated controllability, sometimes under microprocessor control. At least a dozen different external pump devices have been described in the literature.

IMPLANTABLE DELIVERY SYSTEMS

The transition from portable drug infusion systems to implantable drug infusion systems has had interesting parallels with a similar transition about forty years ago from portable pacemakers to implantable pacemakers. The motivations for the transitions are the same. In both cases, portable devices do not provide a complete rehabilitation. The transcutaneous leads and/or tubes cannot be sealed to the skin and always represent an open wound. The patient is always aware of the external device. Also, the external device is vulnerable to mechanical damage. When a patient receives a total implant, the usual response is, "It felt unusual for a few days, but then I forgot about it." Such a response represents as complete a rehabilitation as one could reasonably expect. Early pacemakers required medical attention at frequent intervals, often within a year of implant. Similarly, present implantable drug infusion devices require medical attention at frequent intervals, sometimes weekly or even more often. However, continuing development will certainly produce new and more highly concentrated drugs, larger reservoirs, and improved programming.

The very size and appearance of the portable versus the implantable drug infusion devices remind one of the older portable and implantable pacemakers. The technology to make them and to power them are similar. Manufacturing techniques and quality control measures are all somewhat similar, even though the function of the end device is quite different.

Implantable Pump Designs

Early designers recognized the problems of insulin as a pump medium and first chose to handle simpler materials. Heparin is noncorrosive and easier to pump. Cancer therapy drugs were also easily handled. Anti-arrythmic heart drugs were more troublesome, and insulin began to be successfully handled only very late in the seventies.

By 1983, five implantable pump designs had either seen some clinical evaluation or were nearing that point. P. Blackshear et al. introduced a successful implantable design but did not achieve successful handling of insulin until a decade later.[7] The Pacesetters Company (now Mini Med, Inc.) has claimed their solenoid pump system is more efficient than the peristaltic pump used by others. Siemans/Erlangen has reported on a total implant, again using a peristaltic pump. The Medtronic Company, long a leader in pacemakers, similarly uses a peristaltic pump in their system,[8] which has seen some clinical trials. The first totally implantable insulin system to be implanted in a human on October 25, 1980 was a design by H. Buchwald et al.[9] They later reported five patients with type II diabetes on an implanted pump for a mean of seven months.[10] Their device utilizes a reservoir of fluorocarbon propellant which evaporates at body temperature and maintains pressure against a diaphragm in contact with the drug reservoir. This pump, produced by Infusaid (Model 100), received FDA premarket approval for use in chemotherapy and with heparin. It has also been used to treat diabetes with an Eli Lilly highly purified porcine insulin with 80 percent glycerol and 1 mg/ml $NaHCO_3$ buffer and 0.2 percent phenol. We have designed a programmed microvalve which operates on 3mw of power to meter delivery of drugs from a high-pressure reservoir.[11]

Such pumps provide new horizons to cancer therapy by applying chemotherapy drugs directly to the organ involved. D. McKinstry,[12] W. Ensminger et al.,[13] and A. M. Cohen and Blackshear et al.[14] describe direct continual intra-arterial infusion of FUDR (a cancer drug) to outpatients for hepatic metastasis from colon cancer. The implantable pump avoids surgical incision and permits an outpatient status, marked by improving patient comfort and convenience during long-term chemotherapy.

Sterilization

One last area which we feel has not been adequately addressed is the problem of sterilization of implantable drug infusion systems. From the 1960s to the 1980s, ethylene oxide gas sterilizers largely supplanted both cold sterilization and steam sterilization. However, there is much concern about the safety and effectiveness of gas sterilizers. To be safe and effective, they must be very carefully operated and very carefully maintained. There has been at least one movement to limit the daily exposure time of operators to the machines.

The drug delivery device must be sterilized on the inside as well as on the outside, yet the sterilizing gas is not able to penetrate hard surfaces. Also, the gas must subsequently be thoroughly vented out of any cavities in the device. It does not seem feasible to us to accomplish all this with gas in a daily routine hospital environment.

We suggest that perhaps we must once again look back to the steam sterilizer. This means that all components in the device must be capable of withstanding autoclave temperatures. None of the batteries currently in use meet this criterion, nor do most of today's integrated circuits. Implanted circuit technology has largely derived from pacemaker usage where space is at a premium. In order to build small, pacemaker designers have gone to the use of "Hi K" ceramic capacitors whose parameters unfortunately can be permanently altered by autoclave temperatures. However, autoclavable batteries and autoclavable circuits are within today's scope of technology. We have developed two autoclavable battery systems[15] and have built small infection control modules with one of them. We have autoclaved such modules fifty times without affecting electrical performance. In 1960 we were processing pacemaker transistors for thirty days at 125°C as a quality control measure and that military integrated circuits for operation at 125°C are commercially available. Similarly a number of plastic materials—teflon and silicone among them—can be safely autoclaved. Thus all the components needed for an autoclavable drug delivery system are available today. The problem is not one of research or development but rather one of component selection. One merely needs to put them together and qualify them for implant use.

CONCLUSION

There has been significant progress in the engineering of drugs and drug infusion devices. External (portable) devices are becoming more compact and flexible in operation. Implantable, highly programmable devices that permit outpatient status for many chemotherapy patients are about to become available.

It is not yet possible, however, to take full advantage of the programming capability that can be designed into these devices without two significant steps which remain to be demonstrated*: 1) sensors to permit long-term closed-loop operation; and 2) drugs stable enough for long-term routine use in pumps.

These advances, when and if achieved, will lead to truly significant improvements in patient care through drug administration. They could create a new industry, perhaps approaching the size of the pacemaker industry which has grown from nonexistence to a billion dollar level in this author's professional lifetime.

We are grateful to Max Marsh of Eli Lilly[16] (Indianapolis) and to Henrik Ege of NOVO Industri A/S (Copenhagen) for materials and information relative to insulin production.

NOTES

1. J. Skyler et al., "Biosynthetic Human Insulin: Progress and Prospects." *Diabetes Care* 4, no. 2 (1981): 140.

2. J. Bringer et al., "Prevention of Insulin Aggregation By Dicarboxylic Amino Acids During Prolonged Infusion." *Diabetes* 30 (1981): 83.

3. A. Albisser et al., "Nonaggregating Insulin Solutions for Long-term Glucose Control in Experimental and Human Diabetes." *Diabetes* 29 (1980): 241.

4. D. Schade et al., "Current Status of Portable Insulin Infusion Devices." *Diabetologia* 21 (1981): 425.

5. S. Bessman et al., "The Implantation of a Closed-loop Artificial Beta Cell in Dogs." *Proc. ASAIO*, Anaheim, 1981.

6. H. Broekhuyse et al., "Comparison of Algorithms for the Closed Loop Control of Blood Glucose, Using the Artificial Beta Cell." *IEEE/BME Transactions, BME* 28, no. 10 (1981): 678.

7. P. Blackshear et al., "A Permanently Implantable, Self-recycling, Low Flow, Constant Rate, Multipurpose Infusion Pump of Simple Design." *Surg. Forum* 21 (1970): 136.

8. R. Comben et al., "A Multipurpose Implantable Drug Administration Device and System." *Proc Toronto Intl. Workshop on Insulin and Portable Delivery Systems*, 1982: 54.

9. H. Buchwald et al., "Treatment of a Type II Diabetic Patient By Means of a Totally Implantable Insulin Infusion Pump." *Lancet* 1 (1981): 1233.

10. W. Rupp et al., "The Use of an Implantable Insulin Pump in the Treatment of Type II Diabetes." *New Eng. J. Med.* 307, no. 5 (1979): 267.

11. T. Falk et al., "The Steady State and Pulse Performance of a Solenoid Valve for Use in Drug Delivery Systems." *Proc. Toronto Intl. Workshop on Insulin and Portable Delivery Systems*, 1982: 61.

12. D. McKinstry, "Implanted Drug Delivery Systems for Regional Cancer Therapy." *Research Resources Reporter* (NIH), July 1981: 1.

---

* These two problems, noted in 1983, are still problems in 2000.

13. W. Ensminger et al., "Effective Control of Liver Metastases from Colon Cancer with an Implanted System for Hepatic Arterial Chemotherapy." *ASCO Abstracts*, March 1982: 94.

14. A. M. Cohen et al., "Transbrachial Hepatic Arterial Chemotherapy Using an Implanted Infusion Pump." *Dis. Colon Rectum* 23 (1980): 223.

15. C. Liang et al., "Metal Oxide Composite Cathode Material for High Energy Density Batteries." U.S. Patent 4,310,609, 1982.

16. "Human Insulin from Recombinant DNA Technology" (brochure). April 1982, Eli Lilly.

FOR FURTHER READING

Buchwald, H., et al., "Intra-arterial Infusion Chemotherapy for Hepatic Carcinoma Using a Totally Implantable Infusion Pump." *Cancer* 45 (1980): 866.
Carlson, G., et al., "An Implantable Programmable Insulin Infusion System." *Sandia Report*, SAND 81-2152, 1981.

11

BUT WHAT OF THE FUTURE?

AMERICAN STEWARDSHIP OF THE MOON:
A MILLENNIUM PROJECT

For the future, we foresee (as we did in 1983) that all implantable devices will be autoclavable and MRI-proof. This is a big order, but is achievable.

Also, we would like to extend our vision to other areas, including one that is probably not implantable.

I cannot leave the endeavor of this book without taking a look at the future. My past professional life has largely encompassed electrical power, usually clinically implantable power, but with side excursions into biomass energy and a solar-powered canoe (in which I celebrated my seventy-second birthday by traveling 160 miles on the Finger Lakes of central New York at 3 miles per hour totally under solar power).

In this chapter I would like to expand my sights to global, interplanetary and galactic power for the new millennium. (No one has ever accused me of thinking too small.)

The twentieth century was the century of aviation and the century of globalization. The next century will be the century of space, and in the next millennium globalization will explode into the far reaches of our galaxy. For this I coin the word "Galaxian," with apologies and due credit to Isaac Asimov.

We will be driven by the need for new energy sources. By the year 2050, we will have run out of all the economically recoverable fossil fuels like oil, coal, and natural gas. We will also have run out of places to put the toxic residues of our present nuclear fission reactors. West Valley, New York, doesn't want them, and neither does Nevada. Worse yet, in 2050 all the alternate sources of energy, like hydroelectric, wind, wood, tidal, geothermal, and solar, will not supply even 25 percent of the energy we will need to feed the 10 billion people that will populate Earth by that time. We will have no place to go but nuclear fusion.

Our nuclear fission reactors operate like a slow "A" bomb, splitting heavy plutonium or uranium atoms into smaller elements and giving off power. American and Russian nuclear engineers and physicists have succeeded in slowing down the fission reaction to produce useful power, like Three-Mile Island and Chernobyl, a mixed blessing. Other countries have accomplished this more successfully. France generates a significant part of its energy requirements from fission reactors and has achieved a perfect safety record. Their reactors are all of the same design and are run by nuclear engineers. We build ours all differently and mostly leave the actual operation of the reactors to technicians. But France still has the same problem that we do in the disposal of the toxic residues.

We have never succeeded in slowing down our nuclear fusion reactors, at least not to the point of producing useful power. Nuclear fusion reactors operate like a slow "H" bomb, fusing light atoms like hydrogen or helium. Our present nuclear fusion reactors are classified by the methods used to support the nuclear fusion reaction, which takes place at a temperature much hotter than the surface of the Sun. No bottle on Earth can hold it. The reaction must be suspended by either electromagnetic, electrostatic, or gravitational (inertial) fields.

The TOKAMAK reactor at Princeton, New Jersey, operates by magnetic confinement in a huge 250-ton supercooled electromagnet. The electromagnet exquisitely controls and shapes a magnetic field that physically supports the reaction. The TOKAMAK has never operated longer than a few seconds at a time, and now the federal government has withdrawn its support.

With inertial confinement, hundreds of fantastically powerful lasers are pointed concentrically at a gold capsule containing a small amount of hydrogen. The pressure and the temperature of the capsule are raised to fusion levels and produce a burst of energy. This process must then be repeated—perhaps 100 times per second—to provide a reasonably continuous flow of power. Two such reactors exist in the United States, one in Rochester, New York, and one in Livermore, California. Neither has ever approached "break-even" in power generation.

With electrostatic confinement (Remember picking up paper scraps with a comb which you charged by drawing it through your hair?) the reaction is confined in a 3-foot, 1000-pound spherical vacuum-sealed cage with a very strong electrostatic field inside it. Ions of helium-3 (He-

3) are dropped into the cage and fall through a "polywell" into the electric field where they oscillate backwards and forward at increasing speed until two He-3 ions collide, fusing into an He-4 ion. Two protons are left over from this collision, which come off at a half-million volts of DC electricity which can be directly connected to our existing high-voltage power distribution grids.

Nearly all of our existing power sources are generators that use a heat cycle. This includes our coal, oil, and gas-fired utilities, our automobiles, trucks, and trains, and even our nuclear fission utility power plants. All are "heat engines" and thus are confined to a theoretical efficiency of about 40 percent. Did you know that when you buy a gallon of gas, over 60 percent of the energy you pay for goes out the radiator in the form of waste heat? In fact, that's why you have a radiator in your car in the first place. This is a basic law of physics and there is absolutely nothing you can do about it This is also why our fossil-fueled power utility plants are built by rivers.

But He-3 nuclear fusion reactors are *not* heat engines. They generate electricity directly and are not limited by the "Carnot cycle" efficiency.

More importantly, the He-3 nuclear fusion reactor doesn't generate carbon dioxide or any of the other "greenhouse" gasses. By going to future global He-3 power generation, we can wipe out much of global warming in one fell swoop.

Enough said!

The beauty of this reaction is that the fuel (He-3) is nonradioactive, the process produces no residual radioactivity, and the residue (He-4) is nonradioactive. In fact, the residue, He-4, is what we put in kids' balloons. Thus, He-3 is the perfect fuel.

Does this sound too good to be true? Yes, there are a couple of caveats. The first is that the reaction takes place at a temperature much hotter than the surface of the Sun. But we engineers can handle that. The other is that there is practically no He-3 on Earth. But I tell my engineering students that these are just minor engineering challenges.

He-3 comes to us from the Sun in an ionized form on the solar wind. The ions hit the Earth's magnetic field and get diverted away. They cannot land on Earth, so they drift around and eventually land on the Moon. They have been landing there for four billion years. There is more He-3 energy on the Moon than we have ever had in the form of fossil fuels on Earth. All we have to do is to go there and get it.

There is a tiny bit of He-3 deep in the Earth, from when the Earth was first formed. It comes up to the Earth's surface as a tiny percentage of natural gas. There is a small additional supply of He-3 in our old nuclear bombs in the form of radioactive tritium gas (H-3), which decays into He-3 in about thirteen years (its half-life). Thus, we have enough He-3 on Earth to build one big Earth-bound reactor and one small orbiting reactor. Then we must go to the Moon! My friend and colleague Dr. Gerald Kulcinski, director of the Fusion Technology Institute at the University of Wisconsin in Madison, presently has a reactor running on deuterium-helium, and expects to demonstrate the helium-helium reaction in a few years.[1] We are trying to help him. For years he has operated on a budget of only $35,000 a year, enough for one graduate student. I have long felt that an investment here by the Department of Energy (DOE) of a million dollars a year for the next thirty years would pay a higher return than any other investment this country could ever make.

Most of what I have said here so far is either "le fait accompli," a done deal, or something reasonably achievable with present technology. But now let me dream a little:

He-3 on the Moon is contained in an ore called ilmenite (iron titanate), which contains titanium dioxide. He-3 comes adsorbed on the titanium dioxide. The ilmenite must be scraped off the Moon surface and refined to obtain the titanium dioxide. This will produce by-products of water, carbon, nitrogen, oxygen, and other elements needed to make the manned Moon-colony self-sustaining.

Having little atmosphere or gravity, the Moon-colony could then be an ideal space station from which to blast off for the stars.

The recovered titanium dioxide would then be placed under a large transparent plastic hood and held there two weeks until the Moon rotated around towards the Sun. It will become very hot under the hood and boil off the He-3. Then we would wait two weeks until the Moon rotates around away from the Sun. This would result in very cold temperatures under the hood which would go a long way toward liquifying the He-3. A single shuttle load (about twenty-five tons) of He-3 brought back from the Moon would supply all of the energy needs of the United States for a year.

The cost of the He-3, including the shuttle, the Moon colony, and the ilmenite refinery, amortized over a suitable number of decades, has been calculated to be equivalent to an oil cost of about $8 per barrel of oil. We now pay about $22. The whole project is not only technically feasible, it is economically feasible. In fact, in the opinion of many, including this writer, it is inevitable. There is no reasonable alternative. But if we want to get there by 2050, we had better start now.

Additionally, rocket scientists agree that we have about reached the limit of our ability to travel in space using chemical rockets. To achieve anything near the speed of light we will need a new energy source and a new propellant. Nuclear fission is not an option for galactic travel, but nuclear fusion of light elements like hydrogen or helium would permit approaching the speed of light. To this pragmatic engineer it seems very attractive to refuel your space ships where the fuel is, rather than transporting the fuel to a space station.

History has repeatedly shown that when a new method or material becomes available, new uses for it arise. He-3 is no exception. In only the last few months reports have emerged from Dr. Thomas Daniel at the University of Virginia Health Center and from other sources of the use of He-3 to greatly augment the utility of the magnetic resonance imaging (MRI) procedure in visualizing lung lesions. The patient breathes a few breaths of He-3 that has been superpolarized by laser irradiation. The gas holds this polarization for a few seconds and the resulting polar response is many times more effective than that of the normal water response that the MRI usually sees. This permits visualization of lung lesions down to a resolution of 1mm. When gases are "hyperpolarized," it means a large quantity of the atomic nuclei's "spin"—a magnetic property of quantum particles—point in the same direction. The hyperpolarized gases provide an MRI signal that is about 100,000 times stronger than the signal produced by water, the substance that is normally visualized by MRI scans, according to Dr. Daniel. Physicists Gordon Cates and William Happer at Princeton University, along with Mitchell Albert of Brigham and Women's Hospital in Boston, are primarily credited with the idea of using polarized gases for medical imaging.

Unfortunately the present cost of the He-3 (about $400 per liter) rules it out for routine clinical use, and much effort is going into trying to use the less effective, but cheaper, xenon gas for the purpose. Certainly the availability of reasonably priced He-3 would encourage more research into other possible uses.

So, the challenge of the Moon is clear. The rewards are manifest. But, who should do it?

Only one nation has the equipment, the know-how, and the need for energy to drive this idea forward. That nation is obviously the United States. It needs the same kind of unwavering dedication and the kinds of people that got us the first nuclear submarine and the first man on the moon. We need the kind of leadership exemplified by President Kennedy who ignored the negatives relating to a "man-on-the-moon" and convinced us to "just do it." But we must do it as good stewards, aggressively (but not forcefully) exerting control over the Moon. We can best do this by going there. We are the only nation that has the capability to do it. However, we must exert our stewardship in a generous and altruistic way, making the completed facilities available to all comers, especially including the have-not nations, on an equitable basis compatible with their economies. Also, we must do it soon, while we still have the technological lead to accomplish it, and while the energy shortage is not yet so severe as to encourage terrorist elements (and even our friends) to take extreme steps to block us. Our objective must be not only to alleviate our own energy needs, but also a strong altruism that recognizes that helping to alleviate the world's needs would deter them from extreme and desperate acts if they find themselves with the immediate prospect of *no* energy. In the coming years we must get used to evaluating national and business (and Galaxial) options on a one-hundred-year basis, rather than on a quarterly basis. Procrastination on this item will prove prohibitively expensive in the long run.

It is clear that the nation that assumes stewardship of the Moon now will inherit stewardship of the galaxy in the coming millennium. I think the United States is ready for that challenge. I know I am.

NOTE

1. G. L. Kulcinski and J. F. Santarius, "Advanced Fuels Under Debate." *Nature* 396, no. 24/31 (1998): 724–25.

FOR FURTHER READING

Ashley, R. P., G. L. Kulcinski, et al., "D^3-He Fusion in an Electrostatic Confinement Device." *Proc. 18th IEEE/NPSS Symposium on Fusion Engineering*, IEEE Catalog 99CH37050, 1999.
Farnsworth, P. T., U.S. Patent 3, 358, 402, 1966.

12

CONCLUSION

PARADIGMS

Webster defines a paradigm as "pattern, example, or model." When speaking to groups of young engineers, I have often been asked how one breaks into the mainstream of biomedical engineering. How do you pick your projects, your collaborators, your environment (big business, small business, academic, or government)? In fact, how do you pattern your lifestyle for the happiest results? I have chosen to spend this last chapter on paradigms of design, paradigms of commercialization, paradigms of professionalism, and paradigms of personal motivation.

A Paradigm for Prosthetic Design

When I pick a project on which to work, I don't generally look for a problem to solve. Rather, I look for a place to use something I can do very well. The medical profession is full of problems that are probably insoluble. I have known some engineers in isolated government or big business laboratories who have admittedly made an entire career out of fruitlessly picking away at such a problem. An example is a noninvasive, automatic blood pressure monitor. For decades, dozens of investigators spent millions of dollars looking for a solution and we still do not have one that is good enough to completely replace the cuff and stethoscope. In contrast, one thing engineers can do very well is to make pulses. We do it in radar, in sonar, in computers, and in metronomes. Where can I use a pulse? I can use it to drive a heart. And thus evolves a pacemaker.

What of the design itself? I am a proponent of the "big jump," to throw a breadboard* together and see what it does in the animal lab. What I want is something that works, perhaps not optimally, perhaps only marginally. I'm willing to come back later and fill in the technological details. I may even leave that to someone else.

I generally do not use technicians in my research work. The technician can't see what I see in the oscilloscope. I can't tell him what to look for since I'm generally not sure myself. Conversely, I can't see the problems he has in putting together something I have designed. A simple change that he wouldn't dare to make might vastly improve the manufacturability and the reliability of the device. So, I do it all myself. Confucius said, "He who chops his own wood is twice warmed." I like that.

In an initial design, I always use ridiculously large safety factors. Reliability is exponentially related to safety factor, and it's always easier to cut back on something than to wish you had a little more. Our first 1960 pacemakers had ten mercury cells and delivered an OCV (open-circuit voltage) of 13.5v. We had no idea of what long-term heart stimulation thresholds might be, and we didn't want to be marginal in that critical area. Thus we had few electrode threshold problems in those days.

I never run resistors at more than one-third of their power rating, or capacitors or transistors at more than one-half of their voltage rating. I use only tantalum electrolytic capacitors, Lo-K ceramic capacitors, and the highest quality paper or plastic capacitors. I use only silicon transistors. For batteries, I use only lithium iodine or, more recently, lithium silver vanadium oxide (SVO). Also, I am enthusiastic about some of the newer bromine/chlorine complex (BCX) and sulfuryl chloride batteries for high current pulses. In addition, the lithium carbon monoflouride battery looks quite exciting.

I have a unique method of breadboarding, a first circuit attempt. I draw the circuit on the inside cover of a manila file folder. Then I tape the components on the drawing, adjacent to their drawn symbols. Then I wire everything up, with the battery connector hanging out of the left and the output wires to the right. When a battery is connected to one side and a heart to the other side, the circuit drawing becomes a working pacemaker. I write my test results directly on the other side of the folder when I am finished with my tests, and then I can close up the file folder and drop the whole circuit in my patent file. I have one autoclavable pacemaker pulse generator whose file folder has turned dark brown from repeated bakings at 125°C.

---

*In the 1920s and 1930s circuits were commonly screwed to a wooden breadboard. The term is still used for describing an early prototype.

> ## THE WAY IT WAS
>
> I was called into a recent patent court trial in Minneapolis where the defendant claimed that a patent I had sold to the plaintiff was invalid because the circuit didn't work. I trundled an oscilloscope into the courtroom and connected my patent file folder circuit to it and showed the judge that it did indeed work. That was the last we heard of that.

Certainly, my "loner" approach wouldn't be applicable to all design problems. You couldn't build an atom bomb or a space shuttle that way. But for me, in my little pond, it works fine. If there's any magic to the process, perhaps it's in being able to pick the right device to work on. Some people have the omniscience to look at a device and say, "It's going to go" or "It isn't going to go." I can't explain what goes into such a decision. Fortunately, it only takes one good guess to recoup from half a dozen or more bad ones. The odds are on your side, if you make enough guesses.

Paradigms of Commercialization

Certainly the device must be one that is needed. And this leads to the second principle. If your device satisfies a real need and solves the problem in an eminently satisfactory way, then don't worry about what it costs. If the need was real and you really solved the problem, people will pay the price. Marketing people told us that no one would pay $160 for a ten-year lithium battery when a mercury battery cost only $10. But the need was critical, the lithium battery solved the problem, and we soon found we couldn't make enough of them, even though we expanded our production 300 percent per year for three years.

How do you commercialize a device once you have chosen and built the right one? There are three available paths: 1) build and market it yourself; 2) sell all the rights to someone; or 3) license your rights (and perhaps yourself) to someone who has the means and desire to bring it to fruition.

We have done all three on different occasions. The second is the least satisfying. No one will pay you much of anything for an idea (patented or not) until you have proven that it works and is marketable. If you have gone that far, you probably know enough about the device, the market, and the people in the market to do it yourself.

To build the device yourself, you must either start very small and grow slowly on profits, or you must find financial backing. Don't underestimate the cost and the know-how necessary to set up a manufacturing operation. Aside from startup money, you will need to finance your receivables. It will take about one year from the time you buy your parts to the time you are paid for the completed device. That means you must have about one year's sales available as working capital, just to handle the receivables. For example, if you are fortunate and expand your sales from two million dollars in one year to three million dollars the next, you will have to find a million dollars under some rock, just to carry the receivables, to say nothing of plant expansion and research and development.

The license alternative is an attractive one, but won't last as long as plan one. A license agreement, with minimal up-front money but a good percentage of the gross, is attractive to both licensor and licensee. The licensee can pay his license fees out of profits *after* he has been paid for the device, and the licensor has a strong motivation to really sell the device to the profession and to monitor its quality, because he profits tremendously if it sells well.

Inevitably, however, about ten years later, management will change, the licensee's own research and development people will be restless, and it will be time for the smart licensor to sell all his rights to the licensee and step out.

Another advantage of the licensing option was nonexistent forty years ago. To bring a medical device to market today requires a major investment in time and money that probably only a multimillion-dollar company can afford. From this aspect, a license looks even better.

Another solution is to make only components for devices and not devices themselves. This places the burden and expense of FDA approval on your customer rather than yourself.

I find that the cycle time of bringing a new device to market acceptance is about ten years. We have completed three of these ten year cycles, abandoned three others, temporarily shelved one, and are in the midst of three more. Fortunately some of them overlap, so the sum doesn't exceed my life expectancy.

Don't be afraid of competition from the big companies. On each of our three products that went to successful commercialization, we had to compete against the world's largest electrical manufacturer. We won out in each case, primarily due to a faster response and a more intense attention to device reliability, quality control, and customer service. One of our people said, "If you have to make your drawings before you ship the device, you're too big."

The following represent successful devices we developed. In the 1950s we were approached by the U.S. Air Force at Brooks Air Force Base to supply some ECG amplifiers for the first monkey space flights from

Wallop's Island in Virginia. Their own amplifiers had been designed by one manufacturer and built by another, but were essentially nonfunctional in the final application. In a matter of six weeks, we supplied a new solid-state design which flew successfully on two "Little Joe" flights. We subsequently equipped several more of the air force missions until the space effort was taken over by NASA. We then, as Mennen Greatbatch Inc. (MG Inc.), moved our designs into coronary intensive care theaters, again against competition from the same company. By the late 1960s, MG Inc. (now Mennen Medical Inc.) was number two in the field, second only to Hewlett Packard. The time interval was about ten years.

In 1958 we implanted the first pacemaker, which this book commemorates. We progressed to a proven design and to ten successful patients, and then licensed the device to Medtronic Inc. in 1961. Again, the competition included the aforementioned electrical manufacturer. Medtronic soon filled the marketplace and then moved rapidly through innovative developments and improvements. Ten years later Medtronic was still number one in the field (as they are today), and the two major competitors of the time have ceased pacemaker production.

In 1970 we decided that the most critical need of a pacemaker was a new power source. We began work and saw the first lithium battery implanted in a human in 1972. In the mid-1970s the same large electrical manufacturer announced a new "sealed" mercury battery and an innovative alkali halide battery with a ceramic substrate. Neither ever reached the marketplace. Ten years later nearly all pacemakers had lithium batteries. Not all were ours and not all were lithium iodine, but most were.

What about the failures? We spent five years and a great deal of money (for us, at least) on a bladder stimulator. We thought of the marked benefits of urinary control to a paraplegic. We forgot one thing—the heart is self-excitable tissue, and an impulse applied locally spreads over the whole heart spontaneously. But the bladder is smooth muscle. When one corner is stimulated, only that corner contracts. We used more and more platinum wires and then mesh electrodes and more and more power, without success. Then we went to the sympathetic nerves where they emerge from the spine. After five years, we had two paraplegic dogs that I could make urinate by placing a magnet over the implanted stimulator. Our success rate was about 20 percent and we were told that those nerves in a human are inoperable. So we gave up. Things don't always work.

In chapter 4 we mentioned an atomic battery. It was among the many power sources that we examined as a substitute for the zinc-mercury cells of the 1960s. We studied all the available evidence, much of it contradictory, and decided that the only way was to get in with both feet and see the atomic battery through clinical trials. We collaborated with Hittman Corp. of Columbia, Maryland, and sold all of their output of medical atomic cells to pacemaker manufacturers. After two years and considerable expense, we decided that the atomic battery, although completely safe and effective (Ralph Nader notwithstanding), would never meet acceptance by the medical profession because of the government's restrictive regulatory requirements on the plutonium.

We swallowed our pride and our losses and gave up on nuclear power. Hittman continued on and eventually also gave up after losses considerably greater than ours. As good as it is, the atomic pacemaker never achieved 1 percent of the market. Some things that are technologically fine still don't work out, for nontechnical reasons. At least we tried hard.

Chapters 8 and 9 described bone growth stimulators and electronic control of infection, respectively. We were unable to consistently achieve successful results for these devices. Such devices unquestionably work at some times and don't work at other times. No one really knows why they work or why they don't. As a pragmatic engineer, I'm not happy working in such a void. As a result, we abandoned this work after indifferent results with about fifty implanted stimulators. Recently, considerable interest has emerged in our work and we are now considering renewing our effort, this time on a license basis. Here again, we tried hard, but couldn't put our finger on the key factor to make a clinically consistent device.

And one we shelved.

We have temporarily deferred a project on biomass energy. It involves cloning plants in test tubes in nutrient solutions under "gro-lights." We cloned a hybrid poplar tree which can produce up to seven tons of dry wood per acre per year. When the tree is cut down, it grows right back up from the stump (coppices). If I have two fields of fifteen thousand acres each of these trees, I can cut the fields in alternate years, field-chip them and burn them in turboelectric generators to produce all the electricity for a town of 50,000 people. As any engineer knows, turbines are only 25 percent efficient, taking in high-pressure steam and giving off low-pressure steam. So we will take the low-pressure steam effluent and use it in stills to make wood alcohol for cars. (We successfully ran our old 1967 Dodge truck on 100 percent wood alcohol with a modified carburetor.) The hot water effluent from the stills can be piped in to heat the town. But to get that kind of growth, the poplars need to be very heavily fertilized, so we take the sewage sludge from the town, compost it, and put it on the trees. Thus the whole town becomes energy independent.

We progressed to the point of successfully cloning the trees and have about 40,000 of them planted. We successfully composted two years of sewage sludge from Akron, New York. Remember Confucius's statement about doing work yourself? The first fifteen tons I shoveled with my own hands. That's really getting knee-deep in your work.

THE WAY IT WAS

A Chinese emperor once lined up 5,000 coolies on each side of a sewage lagoon and gave them very long straws with which to blow air into the lagoon. That was the first aerobic digester.

Two events led us to shelve the wood alcohol plan for a time. Our state environmental people would not let us sell our compost to sod growers as we wanted to. Since our company does not accept government financing for research and development, we needed a quick return from at least part of the project. Selling the sludge fertilizer was to be ours. Then, the price of oil fell to the point where we couldn't grow chips profitably. Actually, there should be a law against burning oil. Thirty

---

THE WAY IT WAS

My youngest son Peter drilled out the jets in the carburetor and put on a larger intake manifold. Then we added a two-gallon tank in the cab for alcohol with a transfer valve to change over from gasoline to alcohol. The truck wouldn't start on alcohol so it had to be primed with gasoline first. You squirted gasoline down the carburetor with a squeeze can and held a fire extinguisher in the other hand. My wife wouldn't ride in it! Pickup was marginal but once you got the truck up to speed, it ran just as well as on gasoline. The alcohol stripped the lubrication off the sides of the cylinders so we had to use top lubrication. I added a cup of cooking oil to each gallon of alcohol. When we drove by, the exhaust smelled like burned pancakes. We went through complete regimens of both methanol and ethanol with varying mixtures of water. We were told that water injection would soup up the power, as it did in the fighters in our squadron during World War II. The truck worked best on pure ethanol, nearly as good on pure methanol, and markedly poorer on

(continued)

---

water mixtures, although it would run with up to 30 percent water. We completed our experiments but already felt nostalgic about the truck and didn't want to get rid of it. Fortunately the rusted cab fell clear free of the chassis one day so we could junk the truck in good conscience. If we pick up this project again, we should modify the engine. Alcohol has an octane rating of 120 and should have a very high-compression engine. However alcohol will not "diesel" under any circumstances. So we really should have a diesel engine with a spark plug. Also, we shouldn't use a carburetor. It would be much better to inject heated vapor directly into the intake manifold, mixed with air, or to fuel inject. We learned a lot.

* * *

As an offshoot of our cloning operation, we grew flowers, cactii, raspberries, and woody herbaceous plants for the nursery market. One time we tried cloning roses. Out of fifty, only two grew. One was a white monster with a big green shoot coming up out of the center. The other was a perfect miniature red rose, $1/4$" in diameter, growing in the sealed glass test tube. We entered it in the local garden club flower show and won a prize with it. We decided it had to have a name. Since it was a cloned rose, we called it "Rosemary Cloney."

years from now we'll need all of it to make plastics. If we did that, gasoline would go to $5 per gallon, where it should be. Then we could make wood chips, alcohol, and other alternative fuels profitably. Our alcohol truck experiments were successful, but we were paying $3.50 per gallon for the alcohol. A hollow victory.

Current Projects

We have three projects going on now which are at varying stages of the ten year cycle. One is an autoclavable pacemaker which has about two years of work on it. Another is a collaboration with the Fusion Technology Institute at the University of Wisconsin–Madison involving commercial power from nuclear fusion. The last is a pacemaker which can perform and not be damaged by the intense magnetic field of a magnetic resonance imaging (MRI) procedure.

A Paradigm of Professionalism

The word "profess" has a religious origin. One "professes" one's faith. The engineer should keep this in mind. This derives from medieval days when all knowledge, teaching, and science was in the monasteries. Any interdisciplinary undertaking raises questions about the relative professional standing of its participants from various disciplines. The medical profession has, of necessity, placed its doctors in an exalted position in the hospital hierarchy. Unfortunately, in the past, some doctors place engineers in the status of technicians, as do some technical societies. Fortunately these are in a minority. I personally am a full voting Fellow in the American College of Cardiology, in the British Royal Society of Health, the Institute of Electrical and Electronic Engineers (IEEE), and a full voting member in the North Atlantic Society for Pacing and Electrostimulation (NASPE).

The new teamwork puts much more stress on engineers to perform on a level equal to that of the medical members of the team. Unfortunately, many engineers never rise to this challenge and do indeed act and perform like technicians.

How do we avoid this? First of all, by being true professionals. The biomedical engineer should be an active and contributing member of the engineering society of his own profession, both on the national and local levels. He should strive for the highest member grade to which he is entitled. He should be an active, full member of the biomedical division of his society, and should publish frequently in its journal. He should attend the conventions and personally know the senior people in the field.

Since the biomedical engineer carries a social responsibility to the public (in helping treat patients) I believe he should be a registered professional engineer (PE) in his state.

He should insist on being a coauthor on any publication coming out of his group if he has participated in the work. I carry this one step further and establish, before beginning a project, that medical personnel will publish as senior in medical publications, but that I will publish as senior author when we jointly publish our work in engineering journals. I do not participate in research without such a commitment. When a medical doctor agrees to let you publish as senior author in your journals, you have achieved the equal status that true professionalism demands.

Conversely, you should never allow your name to be used on a paper unless you have studied the paper, have participated in the work, and fully support the paper's conclusions. Your name is your reputation. Your name on the paper means you endorse *both* its medical and engineering conclusions. This, of, course means that you must be knowledgeable enough of that particular medical research area and conversant enough with its language to form a valid, considered opinion about the paper's conclusions. If you can't endorse what your people are saying, you shouldn't be publishing the results.

Be careful about projecting your conclusions beyond what the data support. No one will ever criticize you for saying, "This is what we measured and this is what we saw," as long as your work was carefully and accurately done. Any projections beyond such a statement are risky and should be undertaken only after much thought and discussion.

A Paradigm for Personal Motivation

Ruth Noller and Sid Parnes were organizers of the Creative Problem Solving Institute (CPSI) at the State University of New York College at Buffalo. They taught a five-step process for achieving creativity. It consisted of:

Fact Finding
Problem Finding
Idea Finding
Solution Finding
Acceptance Finding

CPSI was a unique group and I enjoyed being with them. I like their structured approach, too, but I think some of their students sometimes came away with the erroneous conclusion that the above process was a mantra that was all that was needed to be creative. Not so! You have to work.

Each worthwhile thing that I have ever done took about ten years to do. It involved living the project all my waking hours, often with no pay for what I did. The doing was the reward. Being paid, asking for success, and peer approval were all insignificant. At the time I thought such an attitude was crazy. I think now that it is the right way. The good Lord doesn't really care whether you succeed or fail. My most abject failure may be a part of some grand success in His sight that may never take place until long after I'm gone. Thus, I shouldn't fear failure or crave success. To ask for a successful experiment, for professional stature, for financial reward, or for peer approval is asking to be paid for what should be an act of love. I do believe He wants me to try and to try hard, but the reward is in the doing, not in the results. So, I'll never get a swelled head over success or shoot myself over failure because I really don't care. I'll be happy however things go, just for the opportunity to try.

This makes life so much simpler and happier. Without having to fear failure or achieve success, most of life's stresses disappear. I can go ahead and do my work, day by day, not worrying about how much time this book is taking to write when I should be out making money. Rather, I can relax, knowing that I have the finest wife a man could have, five fine kids, and a job I like. I don't have a lot, but I have all I need and no one in the world has anything that I want badly enough to take away from them. Would that the world's leaders could think the same way.

Appendices

CHAPTER 3: ELECTRODES AND LEADS

This chapter was reprinted from material written and published by the author in 1979–1980. Several developments have taken place since 1983. These developments do not, in the author's opinion, justify completely rewriting the chapter, yet they should be acknowledged.

Several new developments and publications relating to carbon electrodes have appeared. The original Richter[1] description of the Siemans/Elema carbon electrode has been augmented by a more recent paper by Elmqvist et al.[2] giving more information and clinical experience with this "activated carbon" electrode.

An excellent paper by Ripart and Mugica[3] describes comparative results, in vitro, with a vitreous carbon electrode (ELA Model PMC), a pyrolytic carbon electrode (Sorin Model S80), against a typical "deep porous" platinum-iridium electrode (CPI Model 4116). We note Ripart's results with carbon, elgiloy, and two platinum electrodes at 1ma and at 8 ma. It is interesting to note that the differences are less marked at the higher current.

Also, we would note a paper by MacCarter et al.[4] that gives additional information on the Amundson porous platinum electrode to which we previously referred.

Lastly we must take note of the tremendous increase in interest in multichamber pacing. Atrial electrodes have improved and physicians have improved their techniques in using them. Many of the objections we raised in the previous pages are becoming less prominent as the decade progresses. We still see a wide gap between the use of multichamber pacing by the "experts" and by local medical centers. There is great concern over the ability of local medical centers to handle the problems that can arise, such as retrograde conduction (positive feedback, in engineering terms). It will be interesting to watch this development.

Notes

1. G. Richter, E. Weidlich, F. Sturm, E. David, G. Brandt, H. Elmqvist, and A. Thoren, "Nonpolarizable Vitreous Carbon Pacing Electrodes." *Proc. VI World Pacing Symp.*, Montreal, 29 (1979): 13.

2. H. Elmqvist, H. Schueller, and G. Richter, "The Carbon Tip Electrode." *PACE* 6, no. 11 (1983): 436.

3. A. Ripart and J. Mugica, "Electrode-Heart Interface: Definition of the Ideal Electrode." *PACE* 6, no. 11 (1983): 410.

4. D. MacCarter, K. Lundberg, and K. Corstjens, "Porous Electrodes: Concept, Technology and Results." *PACE* 6, no. 11 (1983): 427.

CHAPTER 4: POWER SOURCES

Derivation of "ADD" Formula

Measured voltage across a load of R ohms:

Desired voltage across a load of R_x ohms:

$$V = V_{oc} - I_1 R_0$$

$$V_x = V_{oc} - I_2 R_0$$

$$I_1 = \frac{V}{R}$$

$$I_2 = \frac{V_x}{R_x}$$

$$V = V_{oc} - \frac{V}{R}\left(R_o\right)$$

$$\frac{V}{R}\left(R_o\right) = V_{oc} - V$$

$$R_o = \left(\frac{V_{oc} - V}{V}\right) R$$

$$V_x = V_{OC} - \frac{V_x}{R_x}\left(\frac{V_{oc} - V}{V}\right) R$$

$$V_x\left[1 + \frac{R}{R_x}\left(\frac{V_{oc} - V}{V}\right)\right] = V_{oc}$$

$$V_x = \frac{V_{oc}}{1 + \frac{R}{R_x}\left(\frac{V_{oc} - V}{V}\right)}$$

$$\left(\frac{\frac{V}{V_{oc}}}{\frac{V}{V_{oc}}}\right)$$

$$V_x = \frac{V}{\frac{V}{V_{oc}} + \frac{R}{R_x}\left(1 - \frac{V}{V_{oc}}\right)}$$

CHAPTER 5: STATISTICAL EVALUATION OF DEVICE RELIABILITY

Linear Random Failure Analysis

Binomial Approximation

In a random, infinite, linear and undisturbable universe, let p be the probability of a defective unit. Then the probability of a nondefective unit is the complement of p, or:

$$p(0) = (1 - p)$$

The probability of no defective units in a sample of n units is the probability of n individual probabilities, or :

$$p(0/n) = (1 - p)^n \qquad (1)$$

The probability of just one defective unit in n samples is the probability of a defective unit multiplied by the probabilities of nondefective units for all the $(n - 1)$ remaining units in the sample, or:

$$p(1/n) = p(1 - p)^{n-1} \qquad (2)$$

The probability of r defective units in n samples is the probability that r units will be defective and all the rest nondefective. This is:

$$p^r(1 - p)^{n-r}$$

but there are many different ways that this can occur, so we must multiply this by the total number of ways r things can be made from n things. Thus:

$$p(r/n) = \frac{n!}{r!(n-r)!} \; p^r(1-p)^{n-r} \qquad (3)$$

of which (1) and (2) are special cases for $r = 0$ and $r = 1$ respectively.

For n greater than 1,000 r, this reduces to:

$$p(r/n) = \frac{(pn)^r}{r!} (1-p)^{n-r} \qquad (4)$$

with an error of under 0.1 percent.

The probability that 0,1,2,3 . . . up to R units will fail, is the summation of (4) over all values of r from zero to R. Thus:

$$p(R/n) = \sum_{r=0}^{r=R} \frac{(pn)^r}{r!} (1 - p)^{n-r} \qquad (5)$$

$p(R/n)$ is the probability of up to R defective units in the sample. The probability of not reaching R defective units is the complement of $p(R/n)$, or:

$$C = 1 - \sum_{r=0}^{r=R} \frac{(pn)^r}{r!} (1 - p)^{n-r}$$

which is the confidence level of the measurement.

Example 1

What is the confidence level in a failure rate of 0.15 percent per month in a battery after 1,500 failure-free cell-months of exposure?

$r = 0$
$p = 0.0015$
$n = 1,500$

$$P\left(\frac{r}{n}\right) = \frac{(pn)^r}{r!} \qquad (1 - p)^{n-r}$$

$$P\left(\frac{r}{n}\right) = (1)\ (1)\ (.9985)^{1,500} = 0.10522$$

$$C = 1-p\left(\frac{r}{n}\right) = 0.8947 = 89\%\ \text{confidence level}$$

Example 2

If the above exposure is increased to 26,000 cell-months, what is the confidence level in a 0.01 percent per month failure rate?

$r = 0$
$p = 0.0001$
$n = 26,000$

$$P\left(\frac{r}{n}\right) = \frac{(pn)^r}{r!} \qquad (1 - p)^{n-r}$$

$$p\left(\frac{r}{n}\right) = (1)\ (1)\ (.999)^{26,000} = 0.074$$

$$C = 1-p\left(\frac{r}{n}\right) = 0.926 = 93\%\ \text{confidence level}$$

(Note: Example 2 represents the reliability level achieved in WGL 702E/P lithium iodine cell tests as of January 1, 1974.)

Example 3

Let us assume 3,537 cell months of exposure and calculate the confidence levels in a 0.15 percent per month failure rate for 0, 1, and 2 failures:

$p = 0.0015$
$r = 0, 1, 2$
$n = 3,537$

$$p\left(\frac{r}{n}\right) = \frac{(pn)^r}{r!} \quad (1-p)^{n-r}$$

r = 0

$$p\left(\frac{0}{3537}\right) = (1)\,(0.9985)^{3537} = 0.00494$$

$$\therefore C = 99.5\%$$

$$p\left(\frac{1}{3537}\right) = \frac{5.3055}{1!}\,(0.9985)^{3536}$$

r = 1

$$= 5.3055\,(4.9519 \times 10^{-3})^{3537} = 0.2627$$

$$\therefore C = 97.4\%$$

$$p\left(\frac{2}{3537}\right) = \frac{(5.3055)^2}{2!}\,(0.9985)^{3535}$$

r = 2

$$= 14.0741\,(4.9593 \times 10^{-3})^{3537} = 0.06979$$

$$\therefore C = 93.0\%$$

SUMMATION .1010

$$\therefore C = 90.0\%$$

The combined probability that zero, one, or two units will fail is the sum of the individual probabilities. The confidence level that the remainder will not fail is the complement. Thus the confidence level that the failure rate is indeed 0.15 percent per month (one failure in 100 units each 7 months) is 90 percent.

CHAPTER 7: MICROCALORIMETRY

Appendix A

Battery Thermodynamics

The thermodynamics of a battery in an isothermal, constant current environment are best described by the Gibb's free energy equation:

$$H = G + TS$$

where H = the enthalpy or heat content of the reaction, T = absolute temperature, S = entropy (turbulence, randomness), and G = Gibb's free energy.

All of the above are "state" variables, independent of the path of the reaction. Changes are given by:

$$H = G + T\Delta S$$
$$H = nFE_{OC} + T\Delta S$$

where H = a handbook value for the heat of formation, G = a handbook value for Gibb's free energy, $T\Delta S$ is the entropy, irretrievably lost in crystal formation, n = the number of electrons per atom transferred, F = the Faraday constant (96487), and E_{OC} = the open circuit voltage of the cell.

Table 7A–1.
Thermodynamic properties of lithium halides at 300°K

Halogen	Halide	ΔH[a] (Kcal/mol)	ΔG[a] (Kcal/mol)	$T\Delta S$ (Kcal/mol)	E_{OC} (V)
Iodine	LiI	−64.551	−64.450	−0.101	2.795
Bromine	LiBr	−83.870	−81.650	−2.220	3.540
Chlorine	LiCl	−97.578	−91.786	−5.792	3.980
Fluorine	LiF	−147.450	−140.696	−6.754	6.100

[a] From JANAF tables.

The above thermodynamic considerations relate to energy state. However, the microcalorimeter operates on a power (rate of energy flow) basis. To convert, we assume that the cell current remains constant during the measurement period. Then, dividing through by time and converting to electrical units (1μ W/μ A = 23.046 Kcal/mole):

$$P_G = P_H - P_S$$

$$P_G = 2.8009i_L - 0.0044i_L = 2.7965i_L$$

where P is power and i_L is load current. This is the maximum power available to the load of a perfect loss–less cell. In a real cell, this power must be shared with internal I^2R losses so that:

$$P_G = P_0 + P_I + P_L$$

where P_0 = power loss in the source resistance r_0 of the cell, P_I = power loss across marginal insulating materials, and P_L = useful power in the load.

The microcalorimeter sees all these losses except the power in the load. It also sees P_{sd}, the power lost in self-discharge. (This latter is a separate term with its own P_H, P_G, and P_s.) Finally, another heat term must be added; P_C represents exotherm from continuing curing of the plastic materials in the battery. Thus:

$$P_M = P_{sd} + P_S + P_0 + P_C + P_I + P_L$$

$$P_M = P_{sd} + 0.0041 i_L + P_C + P_I + i_L R_L$$

Table 7A–1 lists handbook values of H and G and calculated values of $T \Delta S$ and E_{0C} from Equation 2 for the reaction:

$$Li = \tfrac{1}{2} X_2 - LiX + \Delta H$$

where X represents any halogen going from the elemental state to the crystalline halide state at 300°K (27°C). Note that:

$$T \Delta S = \Delta H - \Delta G$$

and

$$E_{0C} = \frac{G}{nF} = \frac{G}{(1)(96497)} \quad (4.184) = \frac{G}{23.060}$$

Appendix B

Calculation of Enthalpy Power of the LiI Reaction

To calculate P_H we note: 1 mole of LiI = 134 g.

$$\text{Li electrochemical equivalent} \quad = 3.86 \ \frac{AH}{1g \ Li} \ \left(\frac{6.939 \ g}{1 mol \ Li} \right)$$

$$= 26.785 \ AH/mol$$

(1 cal = 4.184 Joules). The battery equation is:

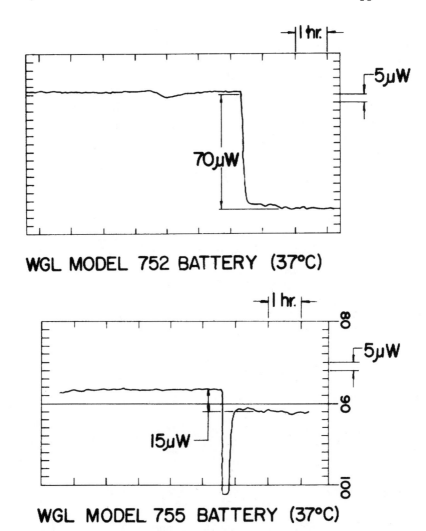

Microcalorimeter readings upon extraction of battery Model 752 and 755 cells.

$$Li = \frac{1}{2}I_2 \rightarrow LiI + 64.551 \; Kcal/mol$$

therefore

$$64.551 \frac{Kcal}{mol} \left(\frac{1 \; mol}{26.785 \; AH} \right) \left(\frac{1AH}{10^6 \; \mu AH} \right) = 2.410 \times 10^{-3} cal/\mu A$$

and

$$2.410 \times 10^{-3} \; \frac{cal}{\mu \; AH} \left(\frac{4.184 \; J}{1 \; cal} \right) \left(\frac{1H}{3,600 \; sec} \right) = 2.8009 \; \mu \; W/\mu \; A$$

which directly gives P_H in terms of load current. Therefore:

$$
\begin{aligned}
1\mu W/\mu A \quad &= \frac{64.551 \; Kcal/mol}{2.8009 \; \mu W/\mu A} \\
&= \frac{(26.785 \; AH/mol)(3.6 \; Ksec/H)}{4.184 \; J/cal}
\end{aligned}
$$

$1\mu W/\mu A = 23.046 \; Kcal/mol/sec$ for LiI

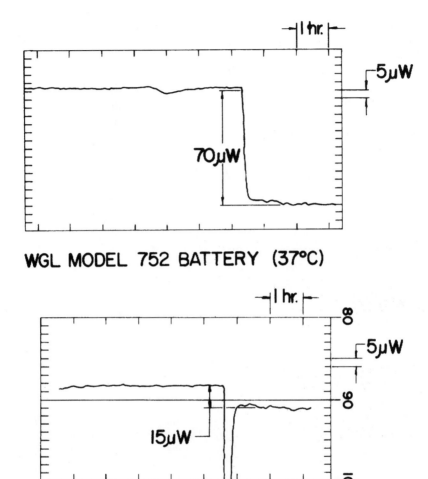

Microcalorimeter readings upon extraction of battery Model 752 and 755 cells.

$$Li = \tfrac{1}{2}I_2 \rightarrow LiI + 64.551 \; Kcal/mol$$

therefore

$$64.551 \frac{Kcal}{mol} \left(\frac{1 \; mol}{26.785 \; AH}\right) \left(\frac{1AH}{10^6 \; \mu AH}\right) \quad = 2.410 \times 10^{-3} cal/\mu A$$

and

$$2.410 \times 10^{-3} \frac{cal}{\mu \; AH} \left(\frac{4.184 \; J}{1 \; cal}\right) \left(\frac{1H}{3,600 \; sec}\right) = 2.8009 \; \mu \; W/\mu \; A$$

which directly gives P_H in terms of load current. Therefore:

$$
\begin{aligned}
1\mu W/\mu A \quad &= \; \frac{64.551 \; Kcal/mol}{2.8009 \; \mu W/\mu A} \\
&= \frac{(26.785 \; AH/mol)(3.6 \; Ksec/H)}{4.184 \; J/cal}
\end{aligned}
$$

$$1\mu W/\mu A = 23.046 \; Kcal/mol/sec \; for \; LiI$$

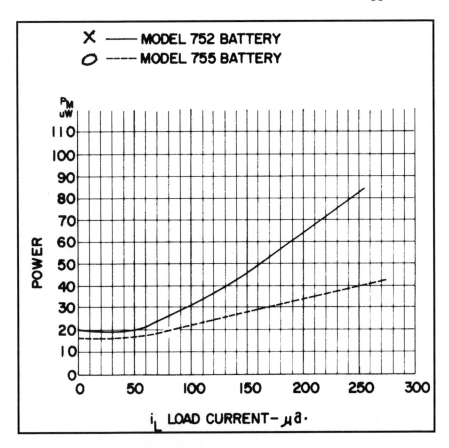

Microcalorimetric power versus battery load current. X=model 752 S/N 14 (1.5 AH).) = 755 S/N 1846 (3AH).

GLOSSARY

ACTUARIAL METHOD: A statistical method of calculating the expected lifetime of devices or people. It was originally developed for the life insurance industry, but was adapted to calculating cancer survival at the Mayo Clinic. Pacemaker people use it to standardize conditions under which pacemaker lifetime is calculated.

ATRIOVENTRICULAR CONDUCTION SYSTEM: The system of nerve nodes and nerve bundles that conduct the "beat" signal from the atria to the ventricles.

BATHTUB CURVE: A curve of failures versus time which looks like a bathtub. The falling portion of the earlier part of the curve indicates failures during the "burn-in" period. Failures along the flat center of the curve are termed "midterm" failures. Failures on the rising terminal portion of the curve are called "wearout" failures.

BISMUTH TELLURIDE: A semiconductor material used in implantable nuclear powered pacemakers to convert the heat from the plutonium[238] nuclear decay into useable electricity to drive the pacemaker.

BLOCKING OSCILLATOR: A circuit often used in military radars to generate short electrical pulses of precise duration. It may be free running or triggered. A free running blocking oscillator with a duration of 1.8 milliseconds and a repetition rate of sixty to seventy minutes was used in the first 1958 pacemakers.

CELL IMPEDANCE: The electrical impedance in ohms of a cell of a battery, typically 10 ohms for a zinc-mercury cell, but as much as 50,000 ohms for an exhausted lithium iodine cell.

CUMULATIVE SURVIVAL ANALYSIS: See *actuarial method.*

CURTAILED LIFETIME: A pacemaker that has been taken out of service for some reason other than pacemaker failure.

ELECTIVE REPLACEMENT: A pacemaker taken out of service at the desire of the physician, for a reason other than pacemaker failure.

ELECTIVE LIFETIME: The service lifetime of a pacemaker electively removed.

ELECTROCHEMICAL POLARIZATION OF PHYSIOLOGICAL ELECTRODES: The buildup of impedance at the surface of a cardiac electrode due to the passage of current across the interface, or passive chemical reactions at the surface.

ELECTROPHYSIOLOGY: The study of the electrical patterns existing on the inner surface of the heart.

ETO STANDARDS: Regulatory standards imposed on the use of ethylene oxide gas sterilizers.

HEART BLOCK: The failure of normal conduction along the auricular-ventricular nerve bundle from the auricles to the ventricles of the heart. This results in a slow heartbeat, or can cause a complete arrest of the heart.

INCOMPLETE LIFETIME: See *curtailed lifetime.*

INSULIN, BIOSYNTHETIC HUMAN (BHI): Human-type insulin made completely from synthetic sources rather than bovine or porcine pancreas.

INTERNAL SELF-DISCHARGE: Battery discharge from internal chemical processes which proceed whether the battery is used or not. This parameter determines the "shelf life" of the battery.

KIETH NEEDLE: A triangular shaped needle with sharp cutting edges which is used to sew skin. In early pacemakers it was used as a percutaneous "Allen wrench" to change the rate or amplitude of the pacemaker output.

LIQUID JUNCTION POTENTIAL/LIQUID MEMBRANE POTEN-TIAL: Electrochemical terms for voltage potentials developed at liquid junctions and membranes of physiological systems.

MICROCALORIMETRY, MICROCALORIMETER, DIFFERENTIAL: Measurement devices that can measure very small temperature differences, as small as the heat generated by a germinating grain of rice. Used here to measure internal self-discharge in batteries.

MYOCARDIAL WIRES: Cardiac pacemaker electrodes in the myocardium (heart muscle).

NUCLEAR HALF-LIFE: The time required for a nuclear isotope to decay to one-half of its original radiation, 2.5 years for promethium, 13 years for tritium, and 87 years for plutonium.

PAVLOVIAN PSYCHOLOGY: A physiological psychology taught by the Russian scientist Pavlov. Its testing methods were widely used in the early U.S. Air Force and NASA animal space shots.

POLARIZATION: See *electrochemical polarization*.

PULSED ELECTROMAGNETIC FIELD: A technique used in early bone-growth stimulators to accelerate the healing of broken bones.

RANDOM LINEAR FAILURE ANALYSIS: A statistical method of predicting device reliability when no failures have yet occurred. It requires the assumption that failures, when they do occur, will be randomly and linearly scattered.

REFRACTORY PERIOD: The period following a heartbeat during which electrical stimulation of the heart will not elicit a response.

SERVICE LIFE: The flat part of the *bathtub curve*.

STERILIZATION, COLD: Sterilization with cold liquid agents such as Clorox. Similar agents were commonly used in early pacemaker work, but now generally replaced with ETO gas sterilization.

STOKES-ADAM SYNDROME: A fainting attack following cardiac arrest from complete heart block.

SYNCHRONY: Synchronous beating between the atria and the ventricles. Results in about 15 percent more maximum cardiac output than nonsynchronous beating.

THORACOTOMY: An open-chest procedure used in early pacemaker days when electrodes were sewed to the outside of the heart. Rarely used since replacement with the transvenous approach.

THRESHOLD, CARDIAC STIMULATION: The voltage needed to elicit a contraction. Threshold rises modestly after implantation, but rapidly in the presence of infection.

TRANSCUTANEOUS: Across the skin into the body.

TRANSVENOUS: Via a vein.

TRANSVENOUS ELECTRODE: An electrode introduced into a neck vein, usually the external jugular vein, and advanced into the ventricle under X-ray observed guidance.

X-RAY BATTERY ANALYSIS: A quality control measure used to estimate the remaining life of early zinc mercury pacemaker batteries and to determine the mechanism of their failure (dendrites and so forth). Not effective for determining the remaining life of lithium batteries, but still used to pick out structural anomalies.

INDEX